700

Natural Health Secrets
Encyclopedia

Published by the Staff of FC&A

FC&A Publishing
103 Clover Green
Peachtree City, GA 30269

Publisher: FC&A Publishing
Editor: Cal Beverly
Production: Cindy B. Eckhart and Laura N. Beverly
Cover Design: Deberah Williams
Printed and bound by Banta Company

Eighth printing August 1992

ISBN 0-915099-30-6

Table of Contents

Aging and Health 1

Weight lifting helps reverse
the weakness of old age 1
Can doctors offer 'fountain of
youth' effect with hormones? 3
Positive outlook on life helps
you age 'gracefully' 4

Alzheimer's Disease 7

New hope for a cure for Alzheimer's disease 7
Ask your doctor about aspirin therapy
for Alzheimer's disease 8

Arthritis 9

Arthritis and aerobics: a healthy combination 9
Commonsense relief from arthritis pain 11
Walking — the aerobic exercise for arthritics 12
If you use a cane, make sure it fits 14

Hot flashes and cold tips for
    relief from aches and pains..............................15
Fish oil supplements provide relief
    from rheumatoid arthritis 17
Put an end to rheumatoid arthritis? 18

Blood Pressure 19

New role for vitamin C: it may
    lower high blood pressure 19
....20
Potatoes and bananas may help
    lower high blood pressure 21
Studies show the benefits of exercise and weight loss in
    controlling blood pressure 22
Could a low-salt diet send your
    blood pressure soaring?...............................24
Job demands influence blood pressure 25
Try bananas or milk to lower
    high blood pressure 25

Breast Cancer....................................27

Breast cancer survival rates nearly
    the same now as 25 years ago 27
Broccoli and brussels sprouts might
    help prevent breast cancer 28
Indulging a sweet tooth may increase
    your risk of breast cancer 30
More news about breast cancer discoveries 32
Radical may not always be better — lumpectomies are just
    as effective..34
Ap - "pear" - ances may be deceiving 35

Upper-body fat may release extra hormones
and trigger cancer growth 36
Body rhythms provide clues
for fighting cancer cells 37
Natural body rhythms play vital role in combatting deadly
cancer cells 38
Soybeans and breast cancer 40
Researchers suspect that electric
blankets increase risk of cancer 41

Breathing and Lung Health 43

Achoo! Yes, it's pollen season again 43
Natural ways to control allergies.....................................45
House dust — an army of allergens 46
You can control dust mites...47
Can asthma be caused by dust mites? 47
Count years — not puffs — when
determining risk of stroke 48
You can turn back the clock on
heart damage from smoking 49
Smoking deadens your sense of smell.............................50
Smoking and depression:
the startling new connection 51
Smoking hides anemia by
producing false hemoglobin 52
Vitamin E and smoking...53
You can stop smoking with
this 13-step system 53
Vitamin C, niacin beat bronchitis....................................57
Take a deep breath to protect yourself
from high blood pressure...57

Breathless? You may be at risk
for a heart attack 58
Keep the cat, not the allergies 59
Man suffers from a lung infection
triggered by chopping firewood 60
Sudden, unexplained coughing?
Check your gloves 61

Cancer 63

Fresh fruits and vegetables help prevent cancer 63
Natural cancer fighting strategies 64
Drink low-fat milk instead of whole
milk to help prevent cancer 67
Dark streak on nail signals cancer 68
Anti-cancer agents are in the spice
cabinet, not medicine cabinet 69

Cholesterol 71

High-fiber cereals for breakfast can
help control cholesterol levels 71
Low cholesterol can be just as
dangerous as high cholesterol 73
Chromium shines as guard against cholesterol 74
Good fat, bad fat 75
It's smelly, but it works 76
Decaf drawbacks 76
Protein and cholesterol 76
Lower blood cholesterol
with psyllium drink 77
Swelling and itching blamed on
allergic reaction to psyllium 78

Colon Cancer 79

Antacid stops 75% of colon cancers? 79

Salty diet linked to colorectal cancer 81

Milk provides essential
    cancer-fighting elements 82

Sitting down to a steak dinner may
    be dangerous for your health 82

Put the starch back into the diet 84

"Skin tags" provide clues for
    detecting colon cancer 85

Dietary fibers differ in
    fighting colorectal cancer 86

Common bean and pea help
    reduce the risk of cancer 87

Diabetes 89

Check your feet for blood sugar disorders 89

Pass the pasta to conserve
    chromium and avoid diabetes 90

Magnesium helps lower blood
    pressure in Type II diabetes 91

New sweetener safe and
    ideal for diabetics 92

Digestive Disorders 95

Do you abuse laxatives? 95

Bananas for indigestion pain? 96

Try iced tea instead 97

Fight the "flu" — loosen up 97

Spice for life 97

Get your head up 98

Relief from diarrhea 98

Can 'harmless' heartburn harm your heart? 98

Treatment helps heal 9 out of 10 peptic ulcers.................100

Drug and Food Reactions 103

Commonly prescribed sedatives
   contribute to falling accidents 103

Side effects of antidepressants could
   be hazardous to your health...104

Treatment for one form of cancer may
   cause another kind of cancer 105

Glaucoma eyedrops may react with
   other prescribed medications.......................................106

Heart medication caution 107

Is microwaved food safe to eat? 108

Stressed out? Put down that coffee cup...............................109

Driving under the influence
   of . . . antihistamines?..110

Products containing sedative-type
   antihistamines 111

Flying high or nose-dive — it's
   all in the medication 112

Name brand or generic — there's
   more at stake than cost alone.......................................113

"Take only as directed..." 114

Check the scale, then check
   the medicine cabinet..114

Blood pressure drugs may trigger diabetes cases............115

Anti-arrhythmic drug side effects may
   defeat the purpose of the drug 116

Ibuprofen: friend or foe? 117

Recurrent NSAID use can result
   in GI complications or even death...............................119

Photocopy blues 119
Beware of mixing drugs 120
And store them safely 121
Don't cool your drugs! 121
Microwaving may contribute
    to food poisoning 121
Feeling dizzy and disoriented? 122
Arthritis drugs cause severe
    kidney damage..122
Anti-baldness drug can cause pain and burning 123
When eating vegetables can be dangerous 123
Alcohol and painkiller combo can damage liver.............124
'Wrinkle cream' responsible for
    nausea, swelling 125
Common ulcer drug triggers
    life-threatening case of diarrhea 126
Acidic foods and drinks reduce the
    effectiveness of nicotine gum................................127
Foods and drinks to avoid
    while using nicotine gum 128
Glaucoma drug causes
    taste disturbances..128
Caution: the medications your doctor
    prescribed might do more harm than good................129
To ensure the safest and most effective
    use of your medicines: Do's and Don't's 132
Drugs that interfere with nutrition.............................133

Exercise and Fitness 135

Regular exercise helps fight
    heart-stopping blood clots 135
Fend off infections with moderate exercise 136

Walk away from cardiovascular disease 137
Personalize your walking time 138
Choosing just the right "equipment" 139
Finding your target heart rate
    and taking your pulse 140
Exercise is a clot buster 141
Flat feet support good news 141
Exercise raises risk of sudden
    death from irregular heartbeats? 142
Reduce the dangers of exercise 143
Start jogging to boost levels of HDL cholesterol 143
Help reduce dizziness with easy exercises 144
Chronic Fatigue Syndrome: exercise
    to get rid of fatigue? 145

Eyesight 147
Caffeine may complicate eye problems 147
Set a date to save your sight 147
Contaminated mascara blinds Georgia woman 149
Vitamins help slash risk of cataracts 150
Sun lovers more prone to cataracts 150
Avoid dangerous look-alikes that
    may cause serious eye injuries 151
Watch the clock for best eye therapy results 151

Health Tips 153
Drink more water to fight confusion 153
Suffering from dry mouth? 154
Aspirin therapy for migraine headaches 155
Re-leaf for headache pain 155
Avoid painful infections easily 156
Change in life-style can create a longer life span 156

Swimmer's ear can spoil summer fun 158
Is man's best friend really his dog? 159
Proper Choice of Pets 164
Life-threatening blood infection
       from deer ticks 165
Pollution slows body's defenses 166
Licorice lovers alert...167
Fast-food flare-up 167
Natural appetite suppressant..168
Tired of puffy eyes? 168
Dieters' blues...169
I beg your pardon 169
Fish and rice 169
Women, count your teeth 170
"Take only at meal times" 170
Milk causes cataracts? 171
Vitamins and nerve damage 171
This 'hot' cream gives pain relief 172
Cool relief for headache pain 172
Are there hidden dangers in your mouth? 173
Painting your walls could poison you 174
Effects of mercury poisoning 175
Aluminum and cast-iron pots and pans are safe...............177
Simple aspirin therapy helps
       prevent migraine headaches 178

Heart Problems 181

Ear crease could be early warning
       sign of fatal heart attack 181
Graze your way to a healthier heart 183
Add fish to your diet to help
       prevent fatal heart attacks..184

Estrogen therapy fights heart disease? 185
Magnesium cuts risk of heart disease 186
Your heart's desire 187
Bigger isn't better 188
'Miracle' clove reduces rates
    of heart attacks 188
Olive oil gives double-barreled
    protection for your heart 189
If your spouse smokes, beware of heart disease 190

Nutrition 191

National Research Council updates RDA values 191
Low-fat diet helps strengthen immune system 193
Fish oil may help prevent the
    development of gallstones 194
Fish oil is not just a passing fad 195
Fish oil — how much is enough? 196
Eat less protein to prevent
    further kidney damage 197
Eat less to live longer 198
Low-fat diet fights heart disease 199
Oat bran extract 200
Raw vegetables help guard
    against cholesterol build-up 201
"It" has long-term benefits 201
Officials hope for 20 percent
    reduction in heart disease 203
Psyllium more effective than oat bran? 203
"Stress" causes cancer? 204
Soup seasoning is good food 206
Unsaturated fats: how do you know
    if they are 'good' or 'bad'? 206

Soybean extract reverses liver disease 208

Osteoporosis 211

Too much salt causes body to lose calcium 211
Osteoporosis affects men
    as well as women...212
Vitamin D helps fight crippling bone loss 213
Drug and vitamin therapy may reverse
    effects of osteoporosis 214
Fluoride fails to prevent osteoporosis 214
Ask your dentist about the risk of
    developing brittle-bone disease 215
Too much caffeine may increase
    your risk of brittle-bone disease 215

Seasonal Affective Disorder 217

Beat SADness and depression
    with light therapy 217
Are you SAD? Here's a list of symptoms 219

Skin Problems.....................................221

Get relief from irritating dry skin problems 221
Tips to relieve dry skin...222
Contact dermatitis: a touchy subject 224
What's causing the itch . . . from
    head to toe 225
A new twist to aspirin pain relief 226
Avoid alcohol if you suffer from psoriasis......................227
Poisonous plants put the itch in summer 228
Delayed allergic reaction to insect stings 229
Vitamin D cream for psoriasis 230
Liver trouble triggers skin disease 231
Gardeners' alert 231

Mask out wart virus 231
Simple remedies for common skin
    disorders among the elderly 232
Check your skin for warning signs: stop
    nutrition problems before they get started.................234

Sleeping Problems 235

Insomnia — the sleeper's nightmare..................235
Falling asleep the natural way 236
Are doctors mistreating sleep problems,
    missing major illnesses?................................237
Skimping on sleep can shorten your life span.................238
Snorer alert — you may be suffering
    from sleep apnea...239
Sleep apnea may be underlying
    cause of some dementia................................240
Getting the most out of your rest.......................241
Fool your body: day and night can
    become just like night and day 243

Strokes 245

Daily aspirin dose could
    reduce your risk of stroke 245
Stroke recovery hampered by some medications.............247
Corn oil is latest weapon in war against strokes.............247

Thyroid Problems 249

Thyroid activity: too much or too
    little can be dangerous................................249
Symptoms of hypothyroidism
    resemble menopause 250

Urinary Problems...............................253

Don't be embarrassed to discuss
   UTI with your doctor...253
Urinary tract infections bring misery
   and possible danger to kidneys...............................254
Urinary incontinence in the elderly 256

Vascular and Circulatory Problems .261

Risk factors for phlebitis and blood clots 261
Exercise decreases risk of blood clots 262
Polycythemia vera 264
Relief from Raynaud's 265
Salt causes brain damage?...266
Vitamin E helps reverse damage
   from hardening of the arteries 267

Vitamins and Minerals.....................269

Blood vessel disease — "B"-ware! 269
Megadoses of slow-release niacin
   could damage your liver..270
More niacin cautions 272
Low selenium levels linked to
   cancers, asthma, digestive ills 272
Pills' crumbling and dissolving
   times are important...275
Severe form of leukemia halted
   with vitamin A drug 276
Vegetarians need vitamins 277
Vitamin E and smoking...277
Vitamin C helps beat drinking problems,
   boosts recovery rate..278
Boost immune response with more vitamin C 279

Women's 2 vitamin deficiencies
  masquerade as deadly leukemia 280
Eat fresh fruits and veggies for proper balance 282
Help prevent loss of hearing
  with vitamin A..283
Vitamin E helps protect arteries from hardening 283
Can vitamins help slow the aging process?.....................284
Beta carotene helps cut
  heart problems in half...285
Vitamin E helps restore muscles
  to healthy state after exercise 287
Vitamin E: who, what, where,
  why and how much?...288

Weight Loss 291

Easy 'OJ diet' might help you lose weight 291
Lose weight to help keep
  your liver in good health 292
More to lose than weight...293
Bouts with gout 294
Diet-and-exercise teamwork 294
Exercise helps you maintain, not lose weight 295
Being too thin may shorten your life span 295
Help reverse drug-induced impotence
  by losing weight 296
Raise resting metabolism rate with exercise 297

Introduction

Natural Health Secrets Encyclopedia is a treasure house of all the latest information about what you can do to improve your health. It tells you how to help prevent or relieve many health problems. It has been written simply to explain some of the fascinating tips that can easily be used for a naturally healthier life.

The editors and publisher of this book have been diligent in attempting to provide accurate health tips that have been confirmed by scientific research. However, this book does not constitute medical advice and should not be construed as such. We cannot guarantee the safety or effectiveness of any drug or treatment or advice mentioned. Some of these tips may not be effective for everyone. Some may work for you but not for other people. Some may work for others but not for you. The only intent of this book is to provide the consumer with easy-to-understand information.

It can be dangerous to rely on self-treatment or home remedies and neglect proven medical treatments. Medical treatment should not be ignored, but natural prevention or treatment may help, too. A good physician is the best judge of what sort of medical treatment may be needed for certain diseases.

With the rapid advances in medicine and health care, we recommend in all cases that you contact your personal physician or health care provider before taking or discontinuing any medications, or before treating yourself in any way.

Best wishes as you strive for a naturally healthier life.

Pleasant words are like a honeycomb,
Sweetness to the soul and health to the
body.

> — Proverbs 16:24

For I will restore health to you,
And your wounds I will heal,
Says the Lord

> — Jeremiah 30:17a

Aging and Health

Weight lifting helps reverse the weakness of old age

Does getting old automatically mean becoming weak, frail and subject to life-threatening falls?

No! says a new study at Tufts University in Boston and reported in *The Journal of the American Medical Association* (263,22:3029).

The secret — weight lifting to strengthen weakened leg muscles.

Ten nursing home residents, ranging in age from 86 to 96, volunteered to pump iron with their legs for eight weeks.

Eight of them had a history of falls, and seven used a cane or other appliance to help them walk. In addition, seven had osteoarthritis, six had heart disease and previous broken bones from osteoporosis (brittle bone disease), and four had high blood pressure.

In other words, most had diseases or disabilities common to the very old.

Each started with about 17 pounds of weight for each leg and progressed to more than 45 pounds on each leg after eight weeks. They exercised three times a week.

During each session, they did three sets of eight repetitions each, with a one- or two-minute rest period between sets.

One repetition is raising and lowering one leg one time. A set is a sequence of repetitions without a rest break.

Despite their frailty, "the average strength gain at eight weeks was 174 percent in the right legs and 180 percent in the left legs," the report says.

Their strength never got stuck on a plateau; it was still on the rise when the weight lifting sessions ended.

"It is likely that at the end of the training these subjects were stronger than they had been many years previously," says Dr. Maria A. Fiatarone, study director.

Not one experienced any falls during or after the weight training, the study says. Only one of the four men dropped out, and that was because he strained an old hernia repair.

But the point of the weight training showed up in improved mobility.

Half of the volunteers were able to confidently walk faster— as much as one-and-one-half times faster than before the leg-weight sessions, the study reports.

Two who had used canes before the weight lifting put their canes away and walked without assistance.

And one of three people who, before the exercise sessions, couldn't rise from a chair without pushing with the arms were able to rise just using the strength in the more muscular legs.

Unfortunately, when the volunteers went back to their old ways of no exercise and sedentary habits, they lost a third of their new-found leg strength within four weeks. That suggests such exercising needs to be continued indefinitely to maintain the benefits.

The weight training caused no problems for those with heart

disease or arthritis, the report says.

Although weight rooms may not become widespread in nursing homes and senior citizen centers, aging experts predict that stretching and movement exercises to strengthen muscles and improve the sense of balance will become common for people even into their nineties.

Since this was an experimental study conducted under strict medical supervision, you should not try similar exercises without checking with your doctor first.

Can doctors offer 'fountain of youth' effect with hormones?

Is the "fountain of youth" pill just months away from your neighborhood pharmacy?

That's the impression you might have gotten from recent news reports of a new synthetic growth hormone.

In the experiments described in the July 5, 1990 *The New England Journal of Medicine* (323,1:1), 12 healthy men ranging in age from 61 to 81 got injections of human growth hormone three times a week for six months.

The results were impressive—the equivalent of reversing 10 to 20 years of aging's effects on lean muscle, spine density and skin thickness, as well as a decrease in fat tissue.

The down side—enough manufactured hormone to produce similar effects would cost you at least $10,000 per year, if you could get some of the scarce stuff.

In addition, some of the men had increased blood pressure readings during their hormone treatments.

Researchers just don't know how long the immediate beneficial effects last, and they don't know whether there are any long-term side effects like increased cancer risks.

Don't look for an "anti-aging" pill to show up in the drugstore any time soon, most scientists advise.

Positive outlook on life helps you age 'gracefully'

The old saying "pretty is as pretty does" may have more truth than we know.

Doctors think that a person's standards of personal cleanliness, grooming and dress actually may tell a lot about her health condition.

Researchers now realize that signs of self-neglect in elderly people are often the first warning signs of hidden illnesses, according to the September 1990 issue of *Senior Patient* (2,9:45).

In other words, a sudden decline in a person's personal care and hygiene may be a warning sign of a health problem or disorder.

For 25 years, the British Red Cross has provided basic "beauty care" to people in hospitals and nursing homes, *Senior Patient* reports. Red Cross workers provide hair, skin and nail care for elderly people. They even help the patients put on fresh make-up and clean clothes.

Such assistance improves patients' self-esteem, fosters a positive outlook on life, and possibly even helps reduce the time it takes for recovery.

Many people may think of the idea as frivolous and too time-consuming. But a little make-up and a fresh hairstyle may actually shorten a person's recovery time in the hospital.

It seems that elderly people who keep a positive outlook on life and continue to keep themselves well-groomed and as youthful-looking as possible are more likely to age more "gracefully" than those who neglect their personal care and hygiene.

Elderly people who try to maintain an attractive appearance through their later years may actually be nurturing their own self-esteem, sense of well-being, social interaction and zest for life.

Alzheimer's Disease

New hope for a cure for Alzheimer's disease

A cure for Alzheimer's disease, a brain disorder that affects the elderly, may be just a few years away, researchers report in *Science* (247,4941:408).

The hope comes in the form of nerve growth factor (NGF for short), a naturally occurring protein that helps keep certain kinds of nerve cells healthy.

Dying nerve cells cause memory loss, one of the first signs of Alzheimer's.

Scientists don't know why brain cells begin to die.

Although NGF can't restore memory and brain function that has already been lost, researchers believe it will help stop further memory loss and brain damage.

They are now reproducing the protein in the laboratory to use in animal studies.

NGF treatment is experimental and hasn't even been tested in humans yet, but researchers say its potential is "very exciting." They also hope to find other proteins as useful as NGF.

Researchers admit there is a risk in trying any new treatment on humans, but the hopelessness of Alzheimer's may outweigh the risk.

As many as four million people in the U.S. have the disease, they say.

Ask your doctor about aspirin therapy for Alzheimer's disease

If you take an aspirin every other day to ward off stroke and heart disease, you may be getting another unexpected benefit as well.

U.S. Pharmacist (15,5:62) reports that some Alzheimer's experts believe that aspirin and the other drugs commonly given for rheumatoid arthritis can prevent Alzheimer's disease.

This theory is only in the testing phase right now. Be sure to check with your doctor before you start taking aspirin regularly.

Arthritis

Arthritis and aerobics: a healthy combination

For many years, doctors told people with arthritis to avoid exercise to help ease their joint pain.

That's changed. Today many doctors recommend just the opposite.

They've found that exercise and increased physical activity seem to improve joint motion and reduce arthritic pain.

Experts stress that aerobic exercise, especially the nonimpact or low-impact varieties, is safe and desirable for arthritis patients, says a report in *The Physician and Sportsmedicine* (18,1:123).

Studies show that aerobic exercise helps produce better heart and lung health. And that helps make a person more self-sufficient, decreases pain and stiffness and leads to improved overall fitness.

Unfortunately, many people with arthritis give up on exercise just because of pain or stiffness in one or two joints. This results in deterioration of the whole body.

People with arthritis should realize that muscle strength actually helps protect weakened joints, researchers say.

Try exercises that use "smooth, repetitive motions such as walking, ice skating, cross-country skiing, and bicycling," recommends Dr. Richard Kyle, chief of the orthopedics department and staff physician for the Arthritis Care Program at Metropolitan-Mount Sinai Medical Center in Minneapolis.

When the weather is bad, go to indoor jogging or cycling machines.

Experts emphasize that some activities should be avoided.

Sports that involve jumping up and coming down hard (basketball, volleyball) may aggravate sensitive joints.

Avoid the risk of joint damage. Proper jogging or walking shoes, for example, are very shock-absorbent and can help cushion arthritic joints.

Help your joints by shedding a few pounds. Losing weight reduces the extra stress on the joints.

A warning — if you've led a sluggish life-style for a while, be careful not to gear up too quickly and thus over-exercise, suggest researchers.

Instead, observe the "two-hour rule." This simple rule says that if you feel pain for two hours after stopping an exercise, you're probably overdoing it.

If this happens, just temporarily scale down the level of exercise, or modify the exercise or equipment in some way.

Be sure to warm up and cool down properly, doctors say. They suggest that you apply light massage and heat or ice as a pain-control measure.

When you exercise also is important.

People with rheumatoid arthritis may need to exercise later in the day due to morning stiffness.

However, people with osteoarthritis who feel worse at the end of the day may need to exercise in the morning.

Be alert to warning signs from your body, experts suggest.

If you experience dizziness, faintness, chest pain, nausea,

extreme joint pain or pain enduring long after finishing the exercises, tell your doctor right away.

If you just dread the thought of exercise, you may find it more enjoyable to exercise with music. Exercising with a friend or with groups of other arthritis patients also makes the experience more fun.

If you're interested in an exercise program, ask your doctor before beginning. Your doctor can help plan a program designed especially to meet your needs and abilities.

Commonsense relief from arthritis pain

You can take the initiative in battling that relentless enemy, osteoarthritis, researchers say.

The first and best weapon against arthritis is a good balance between rest and exercise, says a report in *Senior Patient* (2,1:55).

Getting a good night's sleep, plus morning and afternoon rest periods, helps take pressure off weight-bearing joints and rests tired muscles.

But balance your rest with gentle exercise, experts suggest. Exercise builds muscle strength and helps prevent stiffness and loss of motion.

One of the best forms of exercise for arthritis patients is swimming in a mildly heated pool.

Even if you can't swim, you can still enjoy gentle exercise in the shallow part of a pool, researchers suggest.

Use heat to relieve the pain that comes with osteoarthritis. Try soaking in a warm tub and using a heating pad or hot pack to help ease pain in sensitive joints.

Elderly patients should avoid hot tubs and whirlpools, however, because the water is often too hot.

Gentle massages can also help to relieve those stiff, aching muscles.

Using heat and massage regularly provides great relief from arthritis pain without the extra cost of professional therapy.

One of the best methods of relieving arthritis pain is simply reducing the stress on sensitive joints.

Walkers and properly fitted canes can help improve balance, relieve over-tired muscles and provide stability.

But the cane or walker must "fit" the patient.

A cane or walker that's too tall or too short can magnify arthritic pain and discomfort.

Simple devices in the home can also help ease stress on arthritic joints and improve safety.

To get around better, consider using raised chairs and toilet seats, shower chairs, grab bars in bathrooms and non-slippery rugs and bathmats.

Take away the need to stretch by installing lowered closet shelves and bars.

And replace buttons and zippers with Velcro to ease stress on arthritic hands and arms.

All of these commonsense tips are easy and inexpensive. They're good ways to help relieve osteoarthritis pain and promote more independence in everyday activities.

For more information, contact the Arthritis Foundation, P.O. Box 19000, Atlanta, GA 30326. Ask for their free booklets, "Arthritis: Basic Facts," "Taking Care: Protecting Your Joints" and "Coping With Pain."

Walking — the aerobic exercise for arthritics

You know your heart benefits every time you "take a hike." But did you know that your bones and joints are strengthened as well?

According to *Arthritis Today* (4,3:19), even a moderate walking program can do wonders in reducing joint and muscle stiffness, while actually making bones stronger, denser and less subject to bone-thinning osteoporosis.

Although most people don't realize it, walking is a good aerobic exercise. Dr. James M. Rippe, cardiologist and director of the exercise physiology and nutrition laboratory at the University of Massachusetts Medical School, says that walking, when done properly, is just as beneficial as running or jogging—it just takes longer.

"You don't have to have sweat pouring down your brow to get benefits from aerobic exercise," says Dr. Rippe. "Consistency is more important than intensity."

But don't take that to mean you should "stop and stroll." Try to set a pace that allows you to reach your target heart rate (see article on finding your target rate in the Fitness and Exercise chapter), then maintain it for at least 20 minutes.

People with arthritis often fear exercise will intensify painful flare-ups. The truth is, inactivity causes joints to become stiff and muscles to become smaller and weaker. Walking breaks the cycle of pain and the resulting inactivity.

To loosen stiff joints before walking, try soaking your feet in warm water. Wiggle your toes back and forth as far as they will comfortably move. Dry your feet, dress properly and go for a walk. When you return, soak your feet again, but this time in cool water for about five minutes.

As with any exercise, a warm-up period will increase blood circulation in your muscles, making them more flexible and less likely to suffer from strains, pulls and soreness.

Five minutes of walking slowly should be sufficient. Then pick up your pace, but keep it comfortable, for 10 to 20 minutes.

Do this at least four times a week for a month. Gradually increase your speed, distance and time until you can walk briskly, and continuously, for 30 minutes without feeling fatigued.

Be sure to breathe deeply, in through the nose and out of the mouth. Keep track of your pulse (see instructions) to make sure you stay within your target heart range.

At this point, you are receiving a good aerobic workout. Just remember — if you can't carry on a conversation while you're walking, or you find yourself huffing and puffing, you're pushing too hard.

During the time of an arthritis flare-up, it would be wise to check with your doctor to determine exactly how much exercise is right for you. But even when the walking is somewhat awkward, or you feel limited to shorter walks due to mild pain, the rewards are still definitely worth the effort.

Persons with arthritis report feeling less stressed, and having a better outlook on life due to their daily walks. Walking gives them added flexibility that carries over into other activities and is credited with increasing their lifespan. Not a bad return on a 30 minute investment!

If you use a cane, make sure it fits

Walking canes can do more harm than good if they don't "fit" right. Canes are like shoes — you need to make sure they fit well and are comfortable.

Many patients use canes that are too long. Or they may have the correct size cane, but don't know how to use it properly, says a report in *Senior Patient* (1,2:93).

It's very easy to determine if a cane is the right length. Wear shoes and stand up straight, with your arms hanging loosely at your side. Have someone measure the distance from the crease in your wrist to the ground. This measurement is the best height for the cane, the report says.

Flat, contoured handles at right angles to the cane are better than curved handles (the ones shaped like a shepherd's staff). Flat handles are more comfortable for longer periods of time.

Use flat-bottomed rubber tips for the end of the cane. Rounded rubber tips don't grip the ground as well as tips with flat bottoms.

Remember that rubber tips wear out with regular use just like tires and shoes. They should be replaced occasionally. You can find replacement rubber tips at most drugstores.

Did you know that about half of all cane users hold the cane incorrectly?

They place the cane in the hand on the same side as the painful or injured body part.

The correct way is "opposite" — hold the cane in the hand on the side away from the painful body part.

For example, if your *left* knee pains you, hold your cane in your *right* hand, the report recommends.

Hot flashes and cold tips for relief from aches and pains

Whether you have arthritis or you're a weekend gardener who has overdone a good thing, the correct use of heat or cold therapy can be your ticket to temporary relief from minor aches and pains. *Arthritis Today* (3,3:22) reports that you can gain relief from arthritis pain by using both heat and cold therapy.

Cold therapy temporarily "deadens nerves that carry pain and also reduces swelling and inflammation," states the report. Heat therapy helps relieve stiffness and pain by increasing circulation in the affected area.

Another popular technique used for pain relief is a contrast bath — alternating use of heat and cold.

To get the best results from heat or cold therapy, it's

important to use them correctly. Here are a few tips to help you use heat and cold safely and effectively.

Before using heat or cold:
- Check with your doctor or therapist, especially if you are sensitive to cold or heat.
- Avoid using heat or cold on areas where you have poor circulation or vasculitis.
- Make sure skin is healthy and dry.
- Use extra padding between your heat or cold source and areas where the bone is close to the surface (wrap the heating pad or cold pack in a towel, etc).
- Allow your skin to return to normal temperature between treatments.

During use:
- Avoid using creams, lotions or heat rubs on your skin with heat or cold packs.
- Time yourself. Using heat or cold too long can hurt you. (Ask your doctor about the best length of time for cold or heat therapy.)
- Stay awake, and don't lie on top of the heat or cold pack.
- Remember that a bath or shower that is too hot may make you tired or dizzy.

After use:
- Normal skin will be a uniform pink color. Watch out for warning signs of blisters or dark red or red and white areas.
- Check for any new discoloration or swelling.

Talk to your doctor or therapist about how heat and cold therapy can fit into your overall plan to relieve arthritis aches and pains.

Fish oil supplements provide relief from rheumatoid arthritis

People with active, painful rheumatoid arthritis discovered they had less pain, fewer swollen joints, decreased morning stiffness and improved strength in their hands after taking daily "fish oil" pills for nearly six months.

The daily supplement of omega-3 fatty acids also appeared to halt and even reverse arthritis's invasion of other joints, says the report in *Arthritis and Rheumatism* (33,6:810).

Researchers at the Albany Medical College in New York tried "high" and "low" doses of omega-3 oils on the volunteers.

They gave a third group pills containing olive oil, the report says.

The amounts given were linked to a person's weight.

For example, the "high" dose was the equivalent of a quarter-ounce of fish oil per day for a man weighing 180 pounds, or less than two ounces per week.

Women in the study also got amounts corresponding to their weights.

The "low" dose was half that of the "high."

About one person out of every four of the volunteers experienced fishy after-taste or belching, usual side-effects of taking fish oil capsules.

The researchers suggest that such side-effects are minor compared to side-effects of standard drug therapy for arthritis.

Fish oil supplements can cause increased bleeding times, the report notes.

Those taking the olive oil supplements reported that 24 weeks of vegetable oil failed to ease joint tenderness, morning stiffness or pain levels.

Only the high-dose fish-oil group got significant pain relief, the report says.

The "high-dose" and "low-dose" concepts were defined by the researchers just for the purposes of their clinical trial.

However, other studies have used daily doses of omega-3 oils many times higher than that used in this study, but always with close medical supervision.

Always check with your doctor before taking any supplements, natural or otherwise.

Put an end to rheumatoid arthritis?

A protein produced in the laboratory may soon offer relief to rheumatoid arthritis (RA) sufferers by bringing a certain hormone under control, according to the *Johns Hopkins Medical Letter* (2,2:1).

Too much of the hormone, known as interleukin-1, destroys healthy tissues and leads to pain, swelling and deformity. In animal studies, the protein blocked the production of interleukin-1.

The protein did not repair damage already done but did prevent further damage to healthy tissue. Human studies will begin later this year.

Blood Pressure

New role for vitamin C: it may lower high blood pressure

Doctors one day might tell people with borderline high blood pressure, "Take one vitamin C tablet every day to get your blood pressure back to normal."

That's because researchers have discovered that vitamin C might prevent healthy people from developing high blood pressure and might even help lower slightly elevated blood pressure readings to normal levels, according to a report in *Science News* (137,19:292).

Checking 67 healthy men and women ages 20 to 69, researchers at the Medical College of Georgia in Augusta found that those with high levels of vitamin C in the blood averaged a blood pressure reading of 104/65.

Those with one-fifth those blood levels of vitamin C — but still within acceptable, normally healthy levels — averaged blood pressure readings of 111/73, the report says. The "normal" blood pressure reading usually is considered 120/80.

Researchers suggest that the vitamin somehow pushes blood

pressure down, keeping levels at or below "normal."

That provides a cushion against blood pressure rising beyond healthy levels.

Even people with established high blood pressure may benefit from more C, suggest researchers at Tufts University in Boston.

They checked 241 elderly Chinese-Americans and found the same result: the lower the blood levels of vitamin C, the higher the blood pressure.

Another common thread in both studies: even at the lower ranges of vitamin C measured in the volunteers, none of the people suffered from a vitamin C deficiency.

So the question researchers will be asking is this: are current "minimum" recommended levels of vitamin C (60 milligrams daily) large enough to give this apparent protection against high blood pressure?

Or should people with a tendency toward high blood pressure increase their daily vitamin C intake to around one gram per day, as suggested by U.S. Department of Agriculture scientist David L. Trout?

Check with your doctor first before taking extra vitamin C. Some studies show that taking more than one gram of vitamin C a day can cause kidney stones, gout, diarrhea, cramping and interference with some blood tests.

In addition, suddenly stopping big doses of vitamin C can cause "rebound" scurvy, a serious vitamin deficiency.

You can get vitamin C naturally by eating citrus fruits and dark-green vegetables like broccoli.

Potatoes and bananas may help lower high blood pressure

A low-potassium diet may contribute to high blood pressure, according to a report in *American Family Physician* (41,1:318).

In a recent study, 10 healthy men ate a low-potassium diet or a normal-potassium diet for four to eight weeks.

Those on the low-potassium diet had significantly higher blood pressures after eight weeks than the men on normal-potassium diets, researchers said.

You can add potassium to your diet by eating more fruits and vegetables, such as bananas, beans and peas. Potatoes and potato flour are especially high in potassium.

The estimated minimum daily requirement for potassium is somewhere around two grams, or about one-fourteenth of an ounce.

Other experts urge even higher amounts of potassium for its anti-stroke and blood-pressure-reducing benefits — up to 3.5 grams per day, according to the latest official government recommendation reported in *Recommended Dietary Allowances, 10th Edition* (National Academy Press, Washington, D.C., 1989: page 256).

Earlier studies have shown that a low-potassium diet can also lead to stroke, and researchers plan more studies to confirm their results.

The moral of the story — eat more fruits and vegetables to get more potassium.

If you are taking medicines or suffer from an illness or disease, check with your doctor about how much potassium you should take in each day.

Studies show the benefits of exercise and weight loss in controlling blood pressure

Two recent medical studies praise the benefits of exercise and weight loss in controlling cases of mild high blood pressure.

At the same time, both studies suggest that adding drugs to the exercise and weight loss programs might be just a waste of money, at least in mild cases.

The two natural ways do the job as well as or better than hypertension medicines, according to reports in the *Journal of the American Medical Association* (263,20:2766) and *Medical World News* (31,10:35).

In the *JAMA* report, doctors at three Maryland clinics studied three groups of men with high blood pressure averaging 145/97 mm Hg. All were sedentary, meaning they didn't exercise much, if at all.

They put one group on a beta-blocker drug, propranolol hydrochloride. A second group got a calcium channel blocker, diltiazem hydrochloride. A third group received only a placebo, a fake, harmless pill with no medical effect.

All three groups performed the same kinds of exercises.

Three times a week, all 49 men lifted weights for 30 minutes on a 20-station weight-training circuit. Then they performed 20 minutes of aerobic exercises, either stationary bicycling, walking or jogging.

After 10 weeks, average blood pressure had fallen 14 points systolic and 13 points diastolic, to 131/84, the *JAMA* report says.

More significantly, the drop occurred whether or not the men were taking blood pressure medicine, the report says.

Exercise alone accounted for the improvement, the researchers conclude.

In addition, the men experienced a drop in total cholesterol and LDL ("bad") cholesterol levels.

Levels of HDL ("good") cholesterol increased with the calcium channel blocker but actually decreased with the beta blocker propranolol, the report says.

Added benefits: the men lost a little weight and increased their overall strength by an average of 25 percent.

A second study involved nearly 800 overweight people with mild high blood pressure, according to *Medical World News*.

First, researchers divided the big group into two smaller ones.

They put one of the groups on a diet to lose weight, but let the second group keep eating normally.

Next, they divided each of the two groups into three smaller groups and gave them either a diuretic (chlorthalidone), a beta-blocker (atenolol) or a placebo.

They found that people on the placebo who dropped 10 pounds or more had an average diastolic reduction of 12 points, about the same as those taking blood pressure drugs, the report says.

The catch is this: to get a blood pressure reduction from weight loss alone, you apparently have to lose at least 10 pounds, says Dr. Herbert Langford, chief of hypertension research at the University of Mississippi at Jackson.

Lose less than 10 pounds, and blood pressure remains above normal, the study suggests.

Blood pressure is expressed in millimeters of mercury and measures systolic (upper number) and diastolic (lower number) pressures, as in the "normal" pressure reading of 120-over-80.

Systolic is the pumping pressure of the heart, while diastolic is the at-rest pressure of blood in vessels between heartbeats.

Usually, doctors are more concerned with the diastolic or lower number. Under 90 is considered normal, 90 to 104 is mild, 105 to 114 is moderate, and 115 or over is severe.

Could a low-salt diet send your blood pressure soaring?

For years doctors have been telling you too much salt can send your blood pressure soaring.

Apparently, one doctor has changed his mind.

Dr. Brent M. Egan, a blood pressure specialist, told the audience at the recent annual American Heart Association meeting in New Orleans that a low-salt diet may actually be harmful for some people.

He and his colleagues studied 27 men who were put on a very low-salt diet for one week. They then ate their regular diet for two weeks and then repeated the low-salt diet once more.

Many men with normal blood pressure were "salt-resistant," says Dr. Egan, meaning that their blood pressure did not automatically fall when their salt intake was reduced.

In fact, blood pressure actually increased by as much as five points in some men who reduced salt intake, he reports.

Studies have shown that insulin, a hormone produced by the pancreas, in some cases contributes to hardening of the arteries by helping the body produce excessive cholesterol.

Insulin also encourages the body to retain salt in the kidneys, the report says.

Many men in the study had higher levels of insulin, and Dr. Egan suggests that the body may "adapt" to a low-salt diet by producing more insulin.

The American Heart Association recommends that Americans eat no more than one and a half teaspoons of salt a day. (The AHA has no plans to change that recommendation.)

If you are on a low-salt diet — or if your doctor has recommended one — Dr. Egan suggests that you carefully monitor your blood pressure at home. (You can buy blood pressure monitors at your local drugstore.)

Take your blood pressure every day for one week to establish your baseline measurement before starting the diet. Once on the diet, monitor your blood pressure regularly.

If your blood pressure doesn't fall after one to two months on the low-salt diet, talk with your doctor because, Dr. Egan says, the diet "apparently is not helping."

Job demands influence blood pressure

If you've ever suspected that your high-pressure job is bad for your health, you may have been correct.

According to a study reported in *The Journal of the American Medical Association* (263,14:1929), men who hold jobs with high demands over which they have little or no control are three times more likely to suffer from high blood pressure than men who don't.

These workers are also more likely to suffer from physical changes to the heart that could lead to heart disease over time.

Researchers report that the risk of job-related hypertension increases with age.

Try bananas or milk to lower high blood pressure

High blood pressure? Have a banana!

The solution to mild high blood pressure may be as close as your refrigerator, and as simple as a glass of milk.

Eating foods high in potassium can actually lower your blood pressure, states a report in the *British Medical Journal* (301,6751:521).

Researchers suggest that potassium also protects your heart

by lowering blood cholesterol levels.

Milk, bananas, oranges, vegetables, and meat are all good, natural sources of potassium.

Your doctor or nutritionist can help you plan how to include these foods in your diet to lower your blood pressure.

Breast Cancer

Breast cancer survival rates nearly the same now as 25 years ago

In treating breast cancer, less might be better, suggest two recent reports.

"Physicians are performing less aggressive surgical treatments and finding the survival rates unaltered or sometimes improved," Dr. George Crile Jr. is quoted as saying in *HealthFacts* (15,131:1), published by the Center for Medical Consumers.

Despite vastly better screening methods and improved technology, breast cancer survival rates have remained about the same for the past 25 years, says a study in the April 18, 1990 issue of the prestigious *Journal of the National Cancer Institute* (82,8:693).

The five-year survival rate for all breast cancers was 72 percent between 1965 and 1969, says the *JNCI* report.

The current survival rate has improved by one percentage point, to 73 percent, the journal study says.

Once hailed as a great step forward, chemotherapy for breast cancer "has actually had no measurable impact on survival," says the report in *HealthFacts*.

It quotes a Government Accounting Office (GAO) report to Congress that the five-year survival rate after treatment with chemotherapy stayed around 72 percent between 1975 and 1981.

That is remarkable since in 1975 only about two out of every 10 breast cancer patients received chemotherapy, while nearly seven out of 10 got chemotherapy by 1981.

HealthFacts offers two possible explanations: (1) doctors aren't giving the chemical treatments properly, or (2) "chemotherapy's benefit is modest and possibly not worth the side effects."

Sadly, the number of people still alive seven years after first diagnosis of breast cancer and receiving chemotherapy actually declined 1 percent, from 64 percent in 1975 to 63 percent in 1979, the *JNCI* report indicates.

Most threatened by the steady rise in breast cancer rates: women over 60, says the *JNCI* report.

The same report discounts better screening methods as the reason for a rise in cancer rates.

In other words, there just seems to be more breast cancer than ever before, and new surgical and chemical treatments for it seem not to have helped survival rates.

On the positive side, the figures could be interpreted to suggest that new technology might have kept the survival rates from getting worse as the cases increased.

Broccoli and Brussels sprouts might help prevent breast cancer

You might prevent breast cancer by eating more cabbage, broccoli and other cruciferous vegetables, suggests a new study published in the *Journal of the National Cancer Institute*

(82,11:947).

Scientists are excited about the potential of a powerful cancer-fighting substance discovered in these vegetables.

The substance — indole-3-carbinol — seems to convert one cancer-promoting form of the female sex hormone estrogen into a harmless form.

That harmless form also may block absorption of the "bad" kind of estrogen by breast cells, suggests a report of the study in *Science News* (137,24:375).

The active forms of estrogen have been blamed by many scientists for triggering breast cancer growth.

Anything that blocks active estrogen from breast cells could prevent the formation of cancerous growths, says the *SN* report.

Scientists fed volunteers 500 milligrams of indole-3-carbinol daily for a week.

They used a manufactured form of the natural chemical.

The daily dose was the equivalent of eating about half a head of cabbage a day.

The production of estrogen-blocker jumped by 50 percent after just one week, the study shows.

The results may explain why Asian women — who eat a lot of cruciferous vegetables — have much lower breast cancer rates than American women.

The problem is one of taste — many people just don't like to eat their veggies, especially broccoli and Brussels sprouts.

Dr. Jon J. Michnovicz, one of the researchers who found the cancer fighter, suggests that indole-3-carbinol could be produced in a pill form.

That would allow women who don't like cabbage to take a daily supplement to prevent breast cancer, suggests the report in *SN*.

No such supplement currently exists.

Vegetables containing indole-3-carbinol include cabbage,

broccoli, Brussels sprouts, mustard greens, bok choy, kale, collards, turnip greens and cauliflower.

All these are members of the cruciferous family of vegetables.

The flowers of these vegetables resemble small crosses. Their Latin name means "cross-like."

Several studies have shown that eating a lot of vegetables protects against several other forms of cancer, notably colon and rectal cancers.

But researchers until now had thought the protection came from the fiber contained in the vegetables.

This is the first study to show that a specific natural chemical may be responsible for at least part of the protective effect against breast cancer.

One of every 10 American women will eventually develop breast cancer, according to government statistics.

Slightly more than seven out of 10 women are still living five years after being diagnosed as having breast cancer. Those survival rates have remained about the same for more than 25 years.

Indulging a sweet tooth may increase your risk of breast cancer

A taste for sweet things might be dangerous for women with diagnosed breast cancer, suggest two recent scientific studies.

Eating and drinking foods with high sugar contents produced faster-growing and more deadly tumors in animal tests, report cancer researchers in *Clinical Nutrition* (9,2:62).

Mice fed diets that were high in sugar were nearly three times more likely to die quickly than mice on low-sugar diets, the report says.

Tumors seemed to thrive on sugary diets and were nearly five times as deadly as the same kind of cancerous tumors in mice on a low-sugar diet, reports the journal article.

The researchers found that adding vitamin E and selenium to the diets helped a little bit.

Mice on high-sugar diets that received the two nutrients — known as antioxidants — still developed big, fast-growing tumors, but the tumors were less deadly.

Antioxidants like vitamin E act like scavengers in the blood, neutralizing cancer-promoting chemicals known as oxidants.

The researchers speculate that sugary diets trigger lots of insulin production by the body. Insulin is needed to help body cells use the right amount of sugar.

But insulin also acts like a powerful fertilizer to tumor cells, greatly speeding up the growth of the harmful cells.

The more insulin the body produces in response to a sugary diet, the more fertilizer is poured on cancer cells, the report suggests.

Backing up the suspicions about sugar, a statistical study in the same issue of *Clinical Nutrition* documents a strong link between sugar eating and breast cancer deaths.

Some of the same researchers checked records of average sugar consumption in 20 countries around the world.

Then they cross-checked rates of breast cancer and deaths from breast cancer in those same countries for women between the ages of 55 and 74.

Sure enough, countries with the lowest sugar consumption per person — like Japan and Hong Kong — also have the lowest rates of death from breast cancer, the report says.

Those countries with the biggest hunger for sugar — like the United States and Great Britain — have the highest rates of breast cancer deaths.

The average person in the United States takes in two pounds

of sugar a week, the report says.

But the average Japanese citizen eats less than half that much sugar in a week — 14 ounces on average, the report says.

The report notes that the death rate from breast cancer in Japan is about one-fifth that of the United States.

The statistical comparison took into account and adjusted for other factors, including average daily fat intake, the journal article says.

Underlying both reports is the suggestion that slower-growing tumors result in people living longer after diagnosis of breast cancer.

Based on their findings, the researchers suggest that women with diagnosed breast cancer should cut back on sweets and maintain a low-sugar diet.

More news about breast cancer discoveries

▇ Reviewing 12 big studies about diet and breast cancer, researchers found a strong and consistent link between high-fat diets and increased breast cancer risks among women past menopause.

Eating fruits and vegetables, especially those high in vitamin C, definitely boosts protection against breast cancer, the same review says in the *Journal of the National Cancer Institute* (82,7:561).

▇ If women in North America were to cut their daily consumption of saturated fats to less than one-tenth of their total calories, the breast cancer rate for women past menopause would drop 10 percent, says a report in *Science News* (137,16:245).

Just by eating enough fruits and vegetables to get 380 milligrams of vitamin C daily might drop the breast cancer rate by another 16 percent for all women over age 20, the report says.

That's more than six times the current officially Recommended Dietary Allowance of 60 milligrams. Check with your doctor before taking nutritional supplements.

■ Here's further fuel for the anti-fat argument:

An Italian study found that women who ate lots of meat containing saturated fats were three times as likely to develop breast cancer as women in the same area who got much of their protein from beans, peas and other legumes.

The legume-eaters took in less than 28 percent of their total calories as fats.

Japanese women, who have much lower rates of breast cancer than Americans, get even less fat — usually around 20 percent of their daily caloric intake.

For women in the U.S.A., on the other hand, fats generally account for 38 to 40 percent of our daily calories.

■ Eating more fiber might protect against breast cancer, suggests a study reported in *The American Journal of Clinical Nutrition* (51,5:798).

Scientists studied 24 Seventh-Day Adventist women between the ages of 64 and 83, half of them vegetarians for more than a quarter-century. Other than what they ate, both groups were very similar.

The vegetarians ate more fiber than the other group and had significantly lower levels of estradiol and estrone, two hormones that have been linked to cancerous tumor growth.

Lower levels of these hormones may translate into lower cancer risks, the researchers speculate.

They think that steroid hormones stick to bran fiber, oat hulls, cellulose and lignin and are tossed out of the body quickly.

A high-fiber diet also might protect against endometrial cancers, the report says.

Other studies have shown similar links: eat more fiber and thus lower your risk of breast cancer, according to a review in

Nutrition and Cancer (13,1:1).

■ Eating more fish high in omega-3 fatty acids also might protect women against breast cancer.

Apparently, the omega-3 oils found in deep-water fatty fish help to cut levels of estradiol, a hormone that unfortunately promotes cancer growth.

The fish oil itself also seems to slow down tumor growth, reports a Rutgers University researcher in the *Journal of Internal Medicine Supplement* (225,731:197).

Despite a family history of breast cancer, women past the age of 60 have about the same risk as women with no such history, says a report in *Archives of Internal Medicine* (150,1:191).

The family history risk apparently affects mostly women of child-bearing age.

The longer a woman lives without developing breast cancer, the less likely her heredity will catch up with her, at least in breast cancer risk, the study suggests.

Radical may not always be better — lumpectomies are just as effective

Radical mastectomy is "out," and lumpectomy is "in" as treatment for early-stage breast cancer, according to reports in the *Journal of the National Cancer Institute* (82,14:1180) and *Medical World News* (31,13:31).

A panel of cancer experts agreed that cutting out just the cancerous tumor is usually just as effective as the more extensive surgery.

Sometimes lumpectomy is even better than taking the entire breast and associated tissues in the chest and armpit, the reports indicate.

They noted that relatively few women in the U.S.A. choose

the less-radical lumpectomy, with most still opting for total breast removal.

In the statement prepared for the National Institutes of Health and the National Cancer Institute, the 15 experts suggested that doctors might want to back off from using so much chemotherapy.

Carefully weigh chemotherapy's poisonous side-effects against the sometimes very small benefits of using chemicals to keep the cancer from popping up elsewhere later, they suggest.

Of the 150,000 people who will develop breast cancer this year, about 75 percent of them will have stage one and stage two cancers.

Those are the two kinds for which lumpectomy and follow-up radiation therapy "are as effective as total mastectomy," says the *MWN* report.

Women with ductal cancer of the breast usually choose a total mastectomy, since the cure rate is nearly 100 percent, reports *The Lancet* (335,8688:519).

Ductal cancer usually is confined to one breast and normally doesn't spread beyond that breast, unlike other forms.

They might do as well to choose a less radical option that takes only a quarter of the breast in about three out of four cases, the report suggests.

Ap - "pear" - ances may be deceiving

Better to be a pear than an apple?

Maybe, since a big belly brings a higher breast cancer risk than fatty thighs, say two new studies.

Women past menopause who put on pounds around the middle were nearly twice as likely to develop breast cancer as those who gained weight elsewhere on their bodies, reports Dr.

Rachel Ballard-Barbash in the *Journal of the National Cancer Institute* (82,4:286).

Researchers studying health records of 40,000 Iowa women also found the link between breast cancer and an "apple" shape.

"Pear-shaped" bodies, with fat distributed around the lower hips and thighs, had lower breast cancer rates.

Similar links have been found among body shape, fat distribution and heart attack risks.

Upper-body fat may release extra hormones and trigger cancer growth

Ladies, if you can pinch much more than an inch on your waist, you may have a dangerous amount of upper-body fat.

And the more upper-body fat you have, the greater your risk for developing breast cancer, researchers report in the *Annals of Internal Medicine* (112,3:182).

Losing that fat may decrease your breast-cancer risk, they suggest.

Other studies have shown that being fat increases your risk of breast cancer, but this study is one of the first to show that the location of your fat is even more important.

Luckily, women tend to gain weight below the waistline.

Researchers at South Florida College of Medicine studied 216 overweight women aged 25 to 83 who had breast cancer but had not received hormonal or chemotherapy treatments.

They also kept records on another 600 women without breast cancer.

They measured body fat at the neck, shoulders, arms, waist, hips and thighs.

Women with breast cancer had more fat on the waist, arms, shoulders and nape of the neck than cancer-free women, researchers say.

One of the first signs of breast cancer is a small growth in the breast. Scientists believe "out-of-control" estrogen — a hormone — might trigger breast tissue to begin growing too quickly, resulting in a lump.

Women with upper-body fat have more estrogen and lower levels of hormones that can fight excess estrogen, researchers say.

Upper-body fat may also contribute to gallbladder disease, high blood pressure and diabetes in women, they add.

If you're concerned about your fat distribution and want to lose some weight, talk to your doctor about setting up a safe diet and exercise plan designed especially to meet your needs.

Body rhythms provide clues for fighting cancer cells

An exciting new field of science is just now providing clues to the important roles the body's natural rhythms play in disease treatments and survival times.

In studying chronobiology, scientists are beginning to realize that timing is crucial to the success of breast cancer surgery and chemotherapy, according to a report in the *Journal of the National Cancer Institute* (81,23:1768).

Chronobiologists have discovered that menstrual cycles in women are closely linked to immune system responses.

At least one study shows that there is a good and a very bad time during the menstrual cycle for breast surgery.

They also have found that tumor cells have precise schedules for division and growth, different from normal cells.

Using that growth cycle information, they have been able to

"target" cancerous cells for destruction with chemotherapy while safeguarding normal cells, the journal report says.

While the coordination of treatments with cell division cycles, the circadian sleep-wake cycle and the menstrual cycle holds much promise for potential benefits, most doctors have ignored the new science, the report says.

"The medical establishment... has been rather slow in accepting the discipline, chronobiologists believe," according to the report in *JNCI*.

Natural body rhythms play vital role in combatting deadly cancer cells

The old song, "What a difference a day makes," is especially true in treating breast cancer, new research shows.

The cure rate and survival time after breast cancer surgery depends greatly on when during a woman's menstrual cycle the surgery takes place, according to a new scientific study reported in *The Lancet* (2,8669:949).

The study results imply that survival times and cure rates for other kinds of cancers may hinge on coordinating treatments with the body's natural rhythms.

Women who had breast surgery — both lumpectomy and mastectomy — during or around their menstrual periods had more than four times the rate of recurrence and death, the report says.

On the other hand, women who had their breast cancers removed during days 7 to 20 of the menstrual cycle seemed to have much greater protection against developing another breast cancer or a spread of the disease, says the report.

"The time of resection (surgery) in relation to the menstrual cycle is an independent predictor of the likelihood of future metastatic (spread of) disease," writes Dr. William J.M. Hrush-esky of Albany (N.Y.) Medical College.

He and three other colleagues studied the five-year records of 44 premenopausal women who underwent surgery to remove breast cancers.

Three women were pregnant at the time of surgery, and all three died. Eight of 19 patients who had surgery near or during their periods developed breast cancer again.

Three patients developed new breast cancers plus cancers that popped up elsewhere in their bodies (metastatic cancers). Those three had surgery during or near their periods.

Not a single patient who had surgery between days 8 and 18 of the menstrual cycle developed new or metastatic cancers, the report says.

"Our findings indicate a striking effect of the timing of breast cancer surgery on the incidence and rapidity of disease recurrence and upon disease-free and overall survival," the report says.

The authors speculate that changes in hormone levels in a woman's bloodstream affect the number of natural killer cells in the bloodstream.

That in turn has a great effect on whether the cancer will recur or spread, they believe.

On the basis of both animal and human studies, they believe that a woman's immune system is at a low ebb near and during the menstrual period, possibly to help the egg become implanted in the womb.

During this time, there are fewer killer cells.

On the other hand, a woman's immune system kicks into high gear between days 7 to 21 of the cycle, peaking in the middle, they believe.

A woman has a maximum amount of killer cells flowing in her bloodstream during the mid-cycle, they think.

Those armies of killer cells may be more efficient at mid-cycle at hunting down and killing any cancer cells that escape during surgery, the report indicates.

The study breaks new ground in linking surgery timing and cancer spread to the menstrual cycle.

But it points out a weakness in medical charting and record-keeping by many U.S. doctors and hospitals.

In fact, the study had trouble getting off the ground because of a lack of accurate records. They discovered that many surgeons and hospitals never chart women's menstrual cycles.

"This omission may hinder any attempts to retrospectively study the relation of menstrual cycle to disease and intervention in large numbers of patients," the authors say.

Another implication of this study is that women's menstrual cycles may play a larger than previously suspected role in many disorders, not just breast cancer.

The study cautions that the findings have several limitations, including the small size of the study group.

But the authors have some advice: "We urge doctors to note the date of the [patient's] last menstrual period before any major medical or surgical intervention for any serious illness."

Soybeans and breast cancer

Would eating soybeans several times a week slash your risk of getting breast cancer?

Some researchers suspect that a diet loaded with soybeans may be the reason Asian women have one-fifth the number of cases of breast cancer that American women have, says a report in *The Atlanta Journal* (108,22).

Women of the East eat tofu, or soybean curd, the way we Americans eat eggs and potatoes.

So far, animal tests have raised hopes that soybeans may

provide some powerful cancer prevention, but no tests have been made on people.

Soybeans contain isoflavones, substances that may block some cancer-causing chemicals. The big drawback — soybean products like tofu generally don't win any taste tests.

Researchers suspect that electric blankets increase risk of cancer

Electric blankets may increase your risk of breast cancer, claims a brief report in *American Family Physician* (42,4:1065). Electric blankets produce an electromagnetic field. Prolonged exposure to these electromagnetic fields may increase the risk of breast cancer.

Apparently, the electromagnetic fields somehow lower the amount of melatonin levels in the body. Melatonin is a natural substance in the body that inhibits the growth of cancer cells.

A bit of advice: turn on the electric blanket 15 minutes before you go to bed to warm the sheets. Then turn the blanket off, and pile on the quilts to stay warm.

Breathing and Lung Health

Achoo! Yes, it's pollen season again

For most of us, spring fever means a hammock and a lazy "I'll worry about it tomorrow" attitude.

For millions of people with pollen allergies, however, spring fever means just one thing: Kleenex.

Kleenex for the wheezing and sneezing. The sniffling. The red, itchy, watery eyes.

According to *Health After 50* (2,2:4), pollen allergies are more common in the fall but often last longer in the spring.

In fact, what you may think of as a spring cold may be an allergy. Other allergic symptoms include headache, fatigue, irritability and sore throat.

An allergy is a supersensitivity to "substances that don't bother most people," according to *The Allergy Self-Help Book* (Rodale Press, Emmaus, Penn., 1983). Substances that cause allergic reactions are called allergens.

When you come into contact with any allergen — by touching, tasting or inhaling it — your body's natural defenses spring into action. The immune system releases a flush of histamine to ward off the intruder.

The immune system doesn't break down often. But if it goes haywire and mistakenly targets a harmless substance (such as strawberries or dust), the body releases too much histamine. And it's too much histamine that causes those annoying allergic symptoms.

Generally, allergies develop over time, although you could have an immediate reaction. Often, your body resists the first few encounters with an allergen and then "gives in" to it. (Many people reach their fifties or sixties and wonder why they've "suddenly" developed an allergy to something they've eaten all their lives.)

Although pollen is a notorious allergen (more than 15 million Americans have hay fever), you could be allergic to just about anything. Common allergens include food (such as eggs and wheat), drugs, wool, smoke, dust, pet hair and mold and mildew.

Interestingly, if your parents had allergies, chances are you do too, but not necessarily the same ones.

For some reason, many people choose to "live with" their allergies rather than treat them. However, you have to know what you're allergic to first before you can treat the allergy.

Skin testing is the most common way to test for allergies. Your doctor will inject an allergen just under the surface of your skin, and if a welt appears, you are allergic to that substance.

Skin testing works well in tracking down pollen allergies, but is less successful for food allergies and just about useless for drug allergies (with a few exceptions).

Radioallergosorbent testing is a better allergy detective. RAST is a simple blood test, measuring the amount of antibodies in the blood, which tells your doctor whether your body is trying to fight off an allergen.

Natural ways to control allergies

Knowing you have a pollen allergy doesn't make it much easier to control. Although drugs can help relieve annoying symptoms, specialists agree the best way to control a pollen allergy is to prevent an outbreak in the first place.

Here are some tips from the *Johns Hopkins Medical Letter* :

- Pollen levels are highest between 5 a.m. and 10 a.m., so stay indoors during those hours.
- Keep windows in your home and car closed.
- Keep your home 10 degrees cooler than the outside temperature. A too-cold house can aggravate allergies. Keep your air conditioners and vents clean to prevent dust particles from circulating.
- Keep your lawn mowed short to prevent grass from blooming. Blooming releases pollen into the air.
- Wear sunglasses outdoors to protect your eyes from pollen.
- Don't dry clothes on a clothesline outdoors.
- If you think you've been exposed to pollen, shower as soon as you return home.
- And finally, if you can, take a break from pollen season in your area of the country. A cruise is the ideal choice!

House dust — an army of allergens

If that ball of fuzz under your bed makes you sneeze or wheeze, you may already know that you're allergic...but what exactly are you allergic to?

House dust is made up of lots of different things, and two of the worst offenders are so tiny you can't even see them!

Molds are microscopic plants that live on decaying plant and animal matter in and outside your home. These funguses thrive in warm, moist air.

If you are allergic to funguses, breathing in their airborne spores will cause you to have an allergic reaction. Spores are the "seeds" of the tiny plants.

You can control molds in your environment by following these simple procedures suggested by *Pharmacy Times* (56,5:113):

1. Kill mold in your bathrooms and basement by applying a solution of equal parts water and household bleach.
2. If you must rake leaves and cut grass, use a face mask when you do these chores.
3. Buy an artificial Christmas tree rather than a real one.
4. Store firewood outside instead of inside.

A tougher problem may be getting rid of dust mites.

These tiny relatives of spiders and ticks hide in your upholstered furniture, bedding, curtains and carpets. And they feed on flakes of human skin that you shed every day.

It's not the dust mites themselves that cause your nose to tickle. The trouble comes from the waste products given off by the tiny creatures.

Dust mites' waste products lodge in your furniture or bedding or float through the air in your house, causing some people to have runny noses, asthma or even eczema, a skin problem.

You can control dust mites and molds by keeping the humidity between 30 and 50 percent in your home. It will also help to remove carpeting and to cover mattresses, box springs and pillows with dust-proof cases.

You can control dust mites

There are a few special precautions you can take to control dust mites in your home:

1. Choose washable bedding, not wool or down blankets.
2. Wash all bedding weekly in hot water.
3. Take down heavy curtains and Venetian blinds.
4. Remove carpet.
5. Ask your doctor about Acarosan—a new product that kills dust mites in carpets, beds and upholstered furniture.

Can asthma be caused by dust mites?

New research suggests that some asthma might be caused by childhood exposure to house-dust mites, spider-like creatures too small to be seen with the naked eye.

The mites, which cling to specks of dust in your home, give off a kind of protein called an allergen that triggers allergic responses.

Such exposure possibly could touch off asthma in susceptible people, suggests the study in the Aug. 23, 1990 issue of *The New England Journal of Medicine* (323,8:502).

While the study focused on mites' effect on childhood asthma, the information implies that adults also could be affected so long as they come into contact with dust-borne allergens.

"Over the past 30 years, many of the changes we have made in our houses — such as increased temperatures and the use of fitted carpets, tighter insulation, and detergents effective in cool water — have improved the conditions needed for dust mites to grow," says study author Dr. Richard Sporik.

Count years — not puffs — when determining risk of stroke

Who would you think has the greater chance of stroke — someone smoking 40 cigarettes a day for five years, or the person smoking 10 cigarettes a day for 20 years? Be careful of your answer. You could be dead wrong.

The latest study involving cigarette smokers, as reported by the American Heart Association, reveals new danger associated with the number of years smoking.

Dr. Jack Whisnant, a neurologist from the Mayo Clinic in Rochester, Minnesota, says, "This is the first time that the duration of smoking has been found to be more important in influencing the risk of carotid atherosclerosis than the number of cigarettes smoked over a lifetime."

Carotid atherosclerosis (neck artery disease) is caused by formation of fatty deposits on the walls of the carotid artery, the major blood vessel in the neck that supplies blood to the brain.

Temporary loss of vision or temporary paralysis may be the first signs that the carotid artery is in trouble.

Once the artery becomes completely blocked, or a blood clot

forms, the conditions are right for a stroke.

Dr. Whisnant's study involved 752 men and women who had come to the Mayo Clinic with various symptoms of brain disease and stroke. They took part in a diagnostic technique known as carotid arteriography.

The procedure allows doctors to see the inside of the neck arteries, enabling them to better assess the extent of the damage.

Their medical problems and personal habits, (including smoking, alcohol intake and exercise) were all taken into account.

It was determined that a 60-year-old man or woman who had spent 40 years smoking was 3.5 times more likely to have disease of the neck artery than a nonsmoker, regardless of the number of cigarettes smoked.

The researchers at Mayo Clinic concluded that the length of time spent smoking contributed to neck artery disease more than the actual number of cigarettes smoked, the person's age, or whether or not the person had diabetes or high blood pressure.

Don't just cut back on the number of cigarettes you smoke each day.

According to Dr. Whisnant, this is a "false sense of security."

The only healthy option is to completely stop.

By limiting your smoking years, you could be lengthening your life.

You can turn back the clock on heart damage from smoking

You smoke cigarettes, and you're worried about your health.

But, you won't stop smoking because you think you've already done the damage to your body, and stopping smoking now won't really do you any good.

Well, the good news is that you **can** help your lungs heal if you stop smoking now, even if you have smoked for a long period of time.

The *New England Journal of Medicine* (322,4:213) reports that women who quit smoking greatly reduce their chances of suffering from a heart attack.

By the time a woman celebrates her third anniversary as a nonsmoker, her risk of a first heart attack is no greater than if she had never smoked.

This news is true regardless of how heavy a smoker you might have been, how long you smoked, or where you fit in age in the group of 25-64-year-old women who comprised the detailed study of more than 3,200 women.

Women, rather than quitting, usually are more likely to switch to "low-yield" brands, thinking these brands are safer.

However, "recent evidence indicates that women who smoke low-yield cigarettes have virtually the same risk of myocardial infarction (heart attack) as women who smoke higher-yield brands," the *NEJM* report states.

The study also points out that the risk of a first nonfatal heart attack increases with the amount smoked and is raised considerably for heavy smokers.

The study clearly indicates, however, that the cardiovascular damage is largely reversible within two or three years.

Since you can "turn back the clock" on heart damage, the latest medical advice is this: throw away your cigarettes, allow healing to begin, and in a very few years be free of the heart-abuse caused by smoking.

Smoking deadens your sense of smell

The longer you smoke, the less you can smell, say scientists at the University of Pennsylvania's Smell and Taste Center.

Since the sense of smell affects the taste of food, smokers also may be depriving themselves of many of the pleasures of eating.

The good news: quit smoking, and your sense of smell will return — slowly.

If you've smoked two packs a day for 10 years, it will take about 10 years for your sense of smell to return to the level of a nonsmoker, says the report in the *Journal of the American Medical Association* (263,9:1233).

Smoking and depression: the startling new connection

Doctors have long suspected it, and recent studies now prove that it's true.

People who feel sad and unhappy or depressed day after day, even for months at a time, are more likely to smoke than people who are not depressed, reports the *Journal of the American Medical Association* (264,12:1541).

Furthermore, depressed people have a much harder time giving up cigarettes. In fact, they are 40 percent less likely to be able to quit smoking.

Depressed smokers who do quit find it harder to stay off cigarettes, too.

Researchers suggest that it is hard for depressed people to give up smoking for these reasons:

1. People who are depressed may get hooked on nicotine more easily.

2. Nicotine withdrawal can trigger feelings of depression.

3. And some depressed people who discover that nicotine can lighten their mood use smoking like an anti-depressant medicine

This study serves as a warning for nonsmokers who are depressed: stay away from cigarettes, because you may become chemically addicted to the nicotine more quickly and easily than someone who isn't depressed.

People who smoke and are suffering from depression should consider talking to their doctors about nicotine gum.

Nicotine gum can help you stop smoking without causing the depression of rapid nicotine withdrawal.

Smoking hides anemia by producing false hemoglobin

Feeling tired and worn down? But your doctor can't seem to find anything wrong with you to explain your fatigue and weariness?

It might be because your body has hidden the real problem.

Women who smoke may be suffering from anemia and not know it because the anemia is "masked," warns a recent report in the Sept. 26, 1990 *Journal of the American Medical Association* (264,12:1556). Anemia is a lack of iron in the body.

Apparently, smoking creates an increased level of hemoglobin in the blood.

Hemoglobin is the part of the blood that carries oxygen and iron to the cells in the body.

However, the hemoglobin produced by smoking is a kind of "false" hemoglobin — it doesn't carry oxygen and iron as it should.

So, when your doctor measures the amount of hemoglobin in your body to test for anemia, he sees an increased level of hemoglobin and assumes that you aren't anemic.

But it's the false hemoglobin that he sees. In other words, the false hemoglobin levels could be hiding the lack of good hemoglobin and therefore "mask" your anemia.

So, if you smoke and you feel worn down and tired, ask your

doctor to consider anemia even though your hemoglobin test denies it.

Smoking and lung cancer

You've heard the warnings, and you know the equation: Cigarette Smoking = Lung Cancer.

But now there's a new addition to that equation.

Cigarette smoking can cause more than just lung cancer. It seems that your lungs are no longer the only thing at risk.

Cigarette smoking also can increase your risk of both leukemia and cancer of the bone marrow, reports the Dec. 5, 1990 *Journal of the National Cancer Institute* (82,23:1832).

As with lung cancer, your risk of getting blood or bone cancer increases with the number of cigarettes you smoke daily and the length of time you've been smoking.

The more you smoke and the longer you've been smoking, the greater your risk.

However, there is some good news. Some studies suggest that once a person stops smoking, the body begins a healing process and the chance of cancer decreases.

Even if you've smoked for over twenty years, your body can start healing if you quit smoking.

You can stop smoking with this 13-step system

Even if you are a "hard-core" smoker—someone over age 55 who has smoked for more than 30 years—you *can* stop. All it takes is motivation and a system that replaces old habits with new ones, say researchers in *Senior Patient* (1,5:36). In this report, they detail a system to help older smokers kick the habit.

The system works, the researchers report, and the rewards are great.

A number of studies have shown that older Americans who quit smoking are less likely to develop heart disease and less likely to die from it.

The disease rates "are significantly lower for ex-smokers than for current smokers," researchers say. "And quitting benefits general health and vitality."

Take control

Here's a 13-step system that will allow you to take control of your smoking habit:

(1) "Set a target quitting date." Choose a day you think that stress will be minimal and you won't be around other smokers.

(2) Once you've set a target date, **"keep a record of your smoking habits,** including the times and the places." Keeping a diary will help you recognize how much you smoke and why you smoke. Did a confrontation with a co-worker, rush-hour traffic or an upsetting phone call make you reach for your cigarettes?

(3) Designate a "smoking place" in your home and at work. "Smoke *only* in those places." Choose a place that is inconvenient and uncomfortable. One person chose the corner of his basement; another chose the front lawn. If it's raining or very cold, you might decide to stay indoors rather than smoke. And you will look silly standing there smoking on your front lawn.

(4) Keep ashtrays and lighters only in this designated smoking place.

(5) Don't carry cigarettes with you. Ask nonsmokers (spouse, co-workers) to hold your cigarettes. You will have to ask for a cigarette whenever you want one.

(6) Smoke alone and do nothing else (no watching television, drinking coffee or talking on the phone) while smoking. Take the pleasure out of the habit. Make smoking a chore.

(7) Change smoking postures. If you hold your cigarette in your right hand, switch to your left. If you draw from your cigarette on the left side of your mouth, switch to your right. These changes should make smoking more awkward and uncomfortable for you.

(8) "Buy one pack at a time," and buy lower-tar brands.

(9) "Delay your first smoke of the day and the first one after a meal. Start with a half-hour delay and work up to an hour."

(10) When you want a cigarette, **"put off lighting it for a while.** Hold it in your hand and tell yourself, 'I don't need to light this just yet.'" Once you begin to take control of your habit, the urge for a cigarette might pass.

(11) Set up a support network. Choose sympathetic friends (perhaps ex-smokers) whom you can call when you feel the urge for a cigarette.

(12) Start an exercise program to help prevent weight gain. But remember: Quitting is the goal. You can worry about any extra pounds later.

(13) "Reward yourself often" for accomplishing your goals.

If you cut down smoking before your target date arrives, quitting should be less stressful for you.

If you have cold feet about this, talk to your doctor about prescribing nicotine gum, which will help control the urge to smoke.

Experts stress that you should use nicotine gum to quit smoking — not to cut down — because inhaled nicotine is more potent than the nicotine in chewing gum, and the gum will not work for you.

Cut the caffeine

At the same time you are cutting back on cigarettes, cut back on caffeine as well.

New studies show that smokers trying to kick the nicotine habit tend to load up on coffee and caffeine-containing drinks and foods.

In effect, they increase their caffeine intake to compensate for the loss of nicotine. Doing that makes it harder to quit smoking.

Quitting smoking takes time, especially if you are a long-term smoker.

If your habit gets the best of you the first time, try again—and again. Don't lose your motivation to quit.

Researcher David Dworkin offers these words of wisdom to everyone trying to quit: "No one ever died from quitting smoking."

Vitamin C, niacin beat bronchitis

If you're wheezing from repeated attacks of bronchitis, you may need more vitamin C and niacin, says a digest in *Modern Medicine* (57,10:17).

At the same time, a salty diet may be troubling your lungs. People who ate a tenth of an ounce of salt a day were 27 percent more likely to come down with bronchitis than those on a low-salt diet, the report says.

Take a deep breath to protect yourself from high blood pressure

How deeply you can breathe may determine whether you develop high blood pressure, a startling new statistical study suggests.

Researchers say that the smaller the volume of air you can inhale and exhale from your lungs, the higher your risk of high blood pressure, according to a report in *Science News* (137,25:398).

How much air you can take in and breathe out is called "forced vital capacity."

That and levels of a substance in the blood called uric acid have emerged as possibly "two of hypertension's most predictive risk factors," says the report.

Researchers discovered the early warning signs by examining the detailed medical records of 26,429 people who had been members for at least 18 years of the Kaiser Permanente Medical

Care Program in Oakland, Calif.

People in the upper fifth of uric acid levels were twice as likely to develop high blood pressure by age 55 as the ones in the lowest fifth.

Uric acid is a natural by-product that occurs when the body breaks down old or damaged cells.

Since uric acid can't be further broken down by the body, it must be excreted, usually through the kidneys into the urine.

Shallow breathers were the highest risk group.

The one-fifth with the lowest lung capacity were more than four times as likely to develop high blood pressure as the ones in the upper fifth.

These risk factors stood out even after accounting for the effects of smoking, family history, cholesterol levels and being too fat.

So far, scientists don't know why these two easily measured factors figure so heavily in raising the risks of high blood pressure.

Breathless? You may be at risk for a heart attack

If you are a middle-aged man who is frequently out of breath, you may be a prime candidate for a heart attack, suggests a report in *Modern Medicine* (57,9:139).

In a British study, nearly four out of every 10 men who had breathlessness but no signs of heart disease at their initial screening exam developed angina, suffered a heart attack or died within five years, according to the report.

By contrast, only one out of every 12 men (fewer than one in 10) without breathlessness at screening developed angina or other heart problems during the same period.

Angina is severe pain in the chest and arms brought on by blocked heart arteries. It indicates serious, even potentially fatal, heart disease.

"A strong association was also found between breathlessness and silent electrocardiographic evidence of [coronary artery disease], even in men with no other evidence of [the disease] at screening," say the authors of a report from the British Regional Heart Study, a study involving 7,735 British men 40 to 59 years old.

The likelihood of eventual heart disease seemed to be linked directly to the severity of the breathlessness, the report says.

In other words, the more out of breath you are, the more likely you are to come down with heart problems.

Check with your doctor if even minor exertion causes you to puff and pant for breath.

The doctor may recommend immediate steps you can take to begin lowering your heart attack risk, including changing to a healthier diet and getting into better physical shape.

Keep the cat, not the allergies

Are you tired of the runny eyes, stuffy nose and wheezing caused by an allergic reaction to your house cat?

Or are you dreading your mother-in-law's visits because of her allergic reaction to your house cat?

Don't throw out the cat yet! There may be another solution, says a report in *Science News* (138,7:109).

Researchers have developed a spray that contains tannic acid, a compound found in oak bark, coffee and tea.

Apparently, the tannic acid can chemically alter house dust, pollen, and dust-mite debris so that they no longer cause allergic reactions.

Spraying the tannic acid in carpeted rooms also helps reduce the amount of cat dander in the carpet. The cat dander may be the culprit causing your allergic reactions.

Even if the cat has been gone for a while, the bits of cat fur and skin that remain in the carpet may take several months to die down to tolerable, non-allergic levels. Spraying tannic acid can reduce the dander level to a tenth of its former power.

Tannic acid sprays may be found in pet stores.

A bit of advice: test the spray on a small section of carpet before spraying the whole room to make sure the tannic acid doesn't discolor your carpet.

Man suffers from a lung infection triggered by chopping firewood

Can you catch pneumonia from cutting wood?

A man and his dog both did, reports the Aug. 1, 1990 *Annals of Internal Medicine* (113,3:252).

The 53-year-old Minnesota man spent a day felling a rotten elm tree and cutting it up with a chain saw while his mixed black Labrador played nearby.

Two weeks later, man and dog came down with histoplasmosis, a lung infection triggered by spores of a yeast that grows on rotting wood. Both got well after taking antibiotics.

Places to avoid (or wear a special breathing mask): rotting wood close to streams or lakes, chicken coops, starling roosts, caves, attics and cellars, and any place littered with bird or bat droppings, says the article.

Sudden unexplained coughing?
Check your gloves

Asthmatic reaction triggered by your gloves? Sounds strange, but it could be true if you wear latex gloves while you work.

Several cases of people developing asthma in response to their latex gloves have been reported in *The Lancet* (336,8718:808).

Apparently, the powder on the gloves can trigger an allergic asthmatic reaction. And, the chemicals in the glove itself might also cause the coughing and wheezing that accompany asthma.

Many health care workers and food preparation workers commonly wear latex gloves for sanitary purposes. And many people wear latex gloves around the house when cleaning.

If you develop strange coughing and wheezing, ask your doctor about the possibility of being allergic to your gloves.

Cancer

Fresh fruits and vegetables help prevent cancer

Eating a lot of fresh fruits and vegetables may help you prevent cancer, researchers report in *Food, Nutrition and Health* (13,9: 2).

Fruits and vegetables contain small amounts of acids called phenols, which stop cancer-causing agents from attacking healthy cells.

Where can you find phenols? In almost all fruits and vegetables, but potatoes, grapes and nuts have especially high amounts.

Because phenols are surprisingly plentiful in the diet, scientists say that some people may take in more than one gram every day (although they haven't yet determined the ideal amount).

To get the anticancer benefits, you must eat fresh fruits and vegetables, because processing and storing plants destroy phenols.

Scientists are now looking for ways to "fortify" fruits and vegetables with phenols in the laboratory.

Natural cancer fighting strategies

Many health-conscious readers already know there's a lot of evidence showing that carotenoids (relatives of vitamin A), vitamin A itself, vitamin E, the mineral selenium, omega-3 in fish oil, and dietary fiber seem to protect some people from various kinds of cancers.

But there's more good news about some natural cancer fighters you may not have heard much about.

■ Getting more vitamin D may help people living in areas of high air pollution avoid cancers of the breast and colon, says a report in *Modern Medicine* (57,6:29).

Researcher Cedric Garland says excess sulfur dioxide in the air around industrial cities may block sunlight. Less sunshine means lower levels of vitamin D in the bloodstream.

Lower levels of serum vitamin D are linked with a five-fold increased risk of colon cancer and doubled risk of breast cancer, the report says.

After studying cancer rates in 35,000 men and women in Maryland and 18 Canadian cities, he recommends taking at least 400 IUs (International Units) of vitamin D each day.

That's the same as 10 micrograms (abbreviated either "mcg" or "μg") of cholecalciferol, the chemical name for vitamin D.

Instead of taking it in pill form, Garland's advice is to drink at least four glasses of vitamin D-enriched milk each day. That will give you the 400 IUs, he says.

Of course, as always, check with your doctor before taking any supplements or trying to medicate yourself.

■ Eating strawberries, grapes and Brazil nuts may help your body ward off cell damage from cancer-causing chemicals known as carcinogens, according to researchers at the Medical College of Ohio in Toledo.

Many kinds of nuts and berries contain ellagic acid, says

scientist Gary D. Stoner in *Science News* (133:216).

Ellagic acid snoops out cancer-causing chemicals floating in the bloodstream and neutralizes them, the report says.

In tests on mouse and human lung tissue, the nutty substance also seems to help keep normal cells from becoming cancerous, Stoner reports.

But it only works when added to the system just before or during the time the body is exposed to the carcinogens, the report says.

Supplements of pure ellagic acid don't work well, Stoner says, because the body has trouble absorbing the concentrated version.

The natural stuff, in nuts and berries, is the most easily absorbed form, he says.

■ Cheese, milk and even some kinds of cooked meats — including charbroiled hamburgers — contain a substance that burrows into your body tissue and sets up anticancer guardposts inside the cells themselves, according to researchers at the University of Wisconsin-Madison.

The anticancer substance is a form of linoleic acid, a kind of fatty acid present in large concentrations in cheese and grilled ground beef, says a report in *Science News* (135,6:87).

Linoleic acid is one of three polyunsaturated fatty acids that seem to be very efficient killers of cancer cells, the report says.

But since this form of linoleic acid comes buried in a food's fat — including the saturated kind that can load up your blood with high levels of cholesterol — researchers advise against pigging out on cheese and hamburgers just to get the anticancer effect.

"But within a balanced diet...[linoleic acid] may confer some protection against cancer — particularly when present in combination with other dietary anticancer agents...found in many vegetables, including beans, rice and potatoes," the report concludes.

■ You kitchen veterans will recognize this common spice, easily found at your neighborhood grocery store.

It's the yellow stuff — known as curcumin — found in the spice Turmeric, that seems to halt tumor growth, to prevent new tumors from forming and to hunt down and neutralize cancer-causing chemicals in the blood, says a report in the *Journal of the American College of Nutrition* (8,5:450).

■ Turmeric is peppery and sometimes is substituted for saffron.

It's used in curry recipes, on rice dishes, with yellow vegetables and, in Europe, even as coloring in some beverages like lemonade.

■ Besides being good sources of nutrients, raw broccoli, cabbage, cauliflower and Brussels sprouts also contain cancer-preventing compounds.

But notice that they should be raw, not cooked, say researchers at the University of Manitoba in Winnipeg.

That's because cooking, especially in water, drains the cancer-fighters out of the vegetables, says the report in *Science News* (136,22:351).

These leafy vegetables—members of the Brassica family—contain lots of anticancer compounds called indole glycosinolates.

The compounds prevent breast tumors and precancerous sores inside the stomach in animal tests, the report says.

Indole glycosinolates also trigger release of enzymes that take the sting out of cancer-causing chemicals in some foods we eat, according to the report.

■ By the way, don't use soap to wash your vegetables before eating, warn government health officials.

Soap leaves unseen residues on your vegetables, which can cause intestinal problems, says Myron Johnsrud of the U.S.

Department of Agriculture.

Best way to clean your vegetables: rinse thoroughly under plain running water, says USDA.

■ Several animal studies suggest that diallyl sulfide and other sulfide compounds in garlic fight growth of cancerous tumors in the colon, lung and esophagus (the 9-inch food tube from the mouth to the stomach).

Of course, garlic is well-known as a folk remedy for all sorts of ailments. But there have been very few tests to determine whether its anticancer qualities in animals hold true in people, the report says.

That may change soon. The National Cancer Institute is studying 10 garlic compounds to see if they are safe for human tests.

If they are, and if they prove out in scientific trials, the next step could be "garlic-fortified" cereals, the report predicts.

Drink low-fat milk instead of whole milk to help prevent cancer

"Drink your milk!"

Your mother must have said that at least once every day when you were growing up. And today your doctor still tells you to drink milk because it's so good for you.

But could the kind of milk you drink increase your risk of getting cancer? Researchers in Buffalo, N.Y. think that it could.

According to a report in *Nutrition and Cancer* (13,1&2:89), researchers at Roswell Park Memorial Institute compared the risks of drinking whole milk and the risks of drinking fat-reduced milk (2 percent or skim milk) and found some surprising results.

Their findings show that the fat content of milk is a large risk factor.

Drinking milk with the highest fat content increases cancer risks. Drinking fat-reduced milk appears to protect against many of the same risks.

The study suggested that those who drank large amounts of whole milk were more likely to have cancer than those who never drank whole milk.

And there were fewer cases of cancer among the patients who drank large amounts of fat-reduced milk than among the patients who did not drink fat-reduced milk.

These findings suggest that drinking whole milk may cause cancer, whereas drinking fat-reduced milk may actually help prevent cancer.

Whole milk and fat-reduced milk are both rich sources of calcium, riboflavin, vitamin A and vitamin C.

However, whole milk is the fourth-largest source of calories and the second-largest source of saturated fats in the typical American diet.

Whole milk is also a large source of cholesterol.

Researchers suggest that drinking fat-reduced milk offers all the nutritional benefits found in whole milk without adding the additional fat, calories, and cholesterol from whole milk.

Your best bet: drink fat-reduced milk.

It provides you with vital nutrients without extra fats and cholesterol and helps protect you from the cancer risks that seem to be linked to whole milk.

Dark streak on nail signals cancer

Beware of a black or brown streak that grows from your cuticle toward the tip of a fingernail or toenail. Nail injuries and some medicines will cause nail discoloration, but a dark streak can indicate melanoma, the most dangerous form of skin cancer.

If you notice a dark band growing down one of your finger-nails, see a dermatologist right away. Although nailbed melanoma spreads very quickly to other parts of the body, minor surgery can usually cure this kind of skin cancer when it is detected early.

Anti-cancer agents are in the spice cabinet, not medicine cabinet

That delicious spicy stew that your grandmother taught you to make is not just a yummy meal and a family tradition. It might also be a valuable disease-fighter.

Spices such as ginger, clove, cumin and turmeric appear to have disease-fighting properties, reports the Oct. 25, 1990 issue of *The Atlanta Journal*.

Animal studies show that these spices might help fight cancerous tumors.

But, don't go overboard with the spices. Small amounts are all that is necessary. For example, you don't even need a quarter of an ounce of ginger each day to get the health benefits it provides.

So, continue to season your soups and stews. And now you can enjoy both the taste and the health benefits.

Cholesterol

High-fiber cereals for breakfast can help control cholesterol levels

"Breakfast is the most important meal of the day."

That adage is no longer just motherly advice—it's a medical fact. But not just any breakfast food will do.

Your cholesterol levels throughout the day seem to be directly affected by what foods you choose for breakfast, researchers suggest in the *Journal of the American College of Nutrition* (8,6:567).

A nutrition bonus—adults who "break the fast" with ready-to-eat cereal "have significantly lower fat and cholesterol intakes than those who [eat] other foods at breakfast" or even those who skip breakfast altogether, says the report.

The five-year study, called the National Health and Nutrition Examination, analyzed the food intakes of 11,864 Americans.

To determine whether breakfast really is the most important meal of the day, researchers divided respondents into one of these three categories: (1) cereal eaters; (2) breakfast eaters (but without ready-to-eat cereal); and (3) breakfast skippers.

The non-cereal eaters had the highest fat intakes, followed by breakfast skippers.

Among men and women aged 50 to 74, the study indicates that serum cholesterol levels were lowest for those people eating breakfasts that include cereal and highest for those who skip breakfast altogether.

Additionally, having cereal for breakfast seems to help keep cholesterol levels under control—an important factor in controlling your heart-disease risk.

The breakfast skippers apparently ate higher cholesterol meals later in the day, the study indicates. In addition, they may not have gotten the cholesterol-lowering benefits of a high-fiber meal.

Eating a high-fiber cereal for breakfast can result in weight loss, too, according to a study reported in the *American Journal of Clinical Nutrition* (50,6:1303-1307).

Men and women who eat high-fiber cereal for breakfast tend to feel less hungry throughout the day compared to those who eat other breakfast foods or cereals with low amounts of fiber.

Therefore, high-fiber-cereal eaters tend to eat less food during breakfast and lunch, the report says.

Researchers asked men and women between the ages of 24 and 59 to eat a 7:30 a.m. breakfast of orange juice and cold cereal with milk. They ate either Post Toasties (lowest in fiber), Shredded Wheat, Bran Chex, All Bran or Fiber One (highest in fiber of the five).

Three and a half hours later, they ate a buffet lunch.

The high-fiber eaters consumed about 100 fewer calories at breakfast and about 50 fewer calories at the lunch buffet than those who had eaten lower-fiber cereals, according to the report.

The smaller amount of food consumed at lunch was relatively small, but "theoretically could result in substantial weight loss if continued long-term," the researchers conclude.

By the way, a high-fiber *hot* cereal like oatmeal probably would give many of the same benefits.

Low cholesterol can be just as dangerous as high cholesterol

You've probably heard about the importance of lowering your blood cholesterol levels to avoid possible heart attacks and strokes caused by blood clots.

But is it possible to have cholesterol levels that are too *low*?

The answer, especially if you are over 70, is yes, says a report in *The Lancet* (1, 8643: 868).

Some research indicates that, for some people, extremely low levels of cholesterol in the blood may be just as dangerous — and as deadly — as extremely high levels of cholesterol.

If you are over 70 years of age and have low blood cholesterol levels of 156 milligrams per deciliter (mg/dl) of blood or lower, you have a high risk of a stroke, a French research team suggests.

The "ideal" cholesterol level currently is considered to be 200 mg/dl or below. Any reading above 240 mg/dl is considered excessively high, even dangerous.

A long-term Japanese and U.S. study indicates that extremely low blood cholesterol can actually increase the risk of a fatal stroke known as a cerebral hemorrhage, according to a report in *Science News* (135,16:250).

A cerebral hemorrhage happens when an artery in the brain bursts open.

Cholesterol is an important ingredient in cell walls, and ideal levels of cholesterol help keep cell walls strong and healthy.

Abnormally low blood cholesterol levels weaken cell walls and damage arteries.

High blood pressure puts extra stress on the damaged arteries and may cause a "blowout" — a hemorrhagic stroke.

Another possible factor adding to the high death rate among those with low cholesterol levels may be polyunsaturated fatty acids, the studies suggest.

Older men and women who are on diets to avoid saturated fats may eat large amounts of polyunsaturated fatty acids.

Otherwise good for you, these polyunsaturated fatty acids thin the blood and lower the blood's ability to clot. This greatly increases the risk of a stroke, according to the reports.

If you're concerned about your cholesterol levels, high or low, ask your doctor before you change your eating habits or medicines.

Chromium shines as guard against cholesterol

Chromium does more than just put a bright shine on your car bumper.

One form of this mineral is a vital nutrient that helps your body turn sugars and fats from foods into energy for cells all the way from your brain to your big toe.

New research shows it also might help lower total cholesterol, especially LDL cholesterol, the "bad" type that clogs heart arteries and raises the risk of heart attacks, says a study reported in *The Western Journal of Medicine* (152,1:41).

Researchers at San Diego's Mercy Hospital and Medical Center studied 28 people who ranged in age from 25 to 80.

They tested a supplement called chromium picolinate, a form of chromium that is believed to be easily absorbed by the body. The daily supplements provided 200 micrograms of biologically active chromium.

Among those taking chromium supplements for six weeks, total cholesterol levels dropped 7 percent, and LDL cholesterol (the "bad" form) plunged more than 10 percent.

The chromium supplements also raised by 7 percent the levels of a protein that forms HDL cholesterol (the "good" form).

The researchers suggest that chromium picolinate supplements might help people lower their blood fat levels.

The Recommended Dietary Allowance for chromium is not precise. Instead, the RDA is a range of 50 micrograms to 200 micrograms daily.

Some studies show that the typical American diet provides less than 50 micrograms of chromium per day.

The researchers point out that many people might not be getting enough "bioavailable" chromium in normal diets or even in other forms of chromium supplements.

Adding to their worry is the finding that infection, pregnancy, stress, high glucose intake and just plain aging deplete blood levels of chromium.

Natural sources of chromium include brewer's yeast, calf's liver, American cheese, corn, mushrooms and wheat germ.

Unlike some other mineral nutrients, chromium in its biologically available form appears to be safe even in amounts several times the RDA, and few problems have been reported with chromium overdoses, says the official "bible" of nutrition, *Recommended Dietary Allowances, 10th Edition*, published by the National Research Council (1989: page 242).

As always, check with your doctor before taking any kind of nutritional supplement.

Good fat, bad fat

Watch out for "bad" cholesterol if you have a fat belly or a chubby chest, warns a report in the *New England Journal of Medicine* (322,4:229). Upper body fat, high levels of insulin in the blood and a weakened ability to turn blood sugar into energy seem to work together to lower your level of "good" HDL cholesterol. Less HDL means a worse risk for heart disease, the report says.

It's smelly, but it works

Although many physicians turn up their noses at the very idea, garlic for medicinal purposes is making a comeback, according to *The Lancet* (335:114, 1990).

In recent studies, garlic helped prevent heart disease by lowering "bad" cholesterol, raising "good" cholesterol and keeping blood flowing freely.

The problem is, you'd have to eat much more garlic than you (or anyone living with you) could stand. The good news is that health food stores now sell deodorized garlic in pill form.

Decaf drawbacks

If you drink three to six cups of decaffeinated coffee every day, have your cholesterol checked, recommends *Health Confidential* (4,3:1). Too much decaf can send your LDL cholesterol zooming, putting you at greater risk of heart attack.

Protein and cholesterol

Vegetarians have lower cholesterol levels than meat eaters, and Loma Linda University researchers now know why.

Protein is the key. According to *Stay Healthy* (3,12:46), plant proteins help lower cholesterol, while animal proteins raise cholesterol. These effects occur no matter what type of fat a person consumes.

Lower blood cholesterol with psyllium drink

It's cheap. It's easy to get. And it lowers cholesterol. The "it" is psyllium.

A recent study on the cholesterol-lowering effects of psyllium showed that psyllium lowers both total cholesterol levels and LDL cholesterol levels, says the *Southern Medical Journal* (83,10:1131).

The people who volunteered for the study took psyllium twice daily. They mixed three packets of instant Metamucil into a 12-ounce glass of water. (Metamucil contains psyllium.) The volunteers each drank one glass of Metamucil before breakfast and one after dinner. They also drank a 12-ounce glass of water after each glass of Metamucil.

The volunteers also participated in the American Heart Association diet while they tested the psyllium. The AHA diet helps promote good health by lowering weight and cholesterol levels.

Researchers suggest that psyllium is probably most effective in lowering cholesterol when it is combined with the American Heart Association diet. (You can contact the American Heart Association for a copy of this diet.)

The combination of the AHA diet and the psyllium drinks resulted in a 17.3 percent decrease in total cholesterol in men and a 7.7 percent decrease in total cholesterol in women.

The study also showed a 20 percent decrease in LDL cholesterol in men and an 11.6 decrease in LDL cholesterol in women.

The lower cholesterol levels help promote good health and

help protect people from heart disease.

If you're interested in lowering your cholesterol using psyllium, contact your doctor. Some people are allergic to psyllium, and they can have serious reactions.

Swelling and itching blamed on allergic reaction to psyllium

Psyllium is great for lowering cholesterol — if you're not allergic to it, that is.

But some people are allergic to psyllium.

Recently, a 43-year-old woman had to see a doctor because of an allergic reaction she had to the psyllium contained in the cereal, Heartwise, reports the *New England Journal of Medicine* (323,15:1072).

The woman developed swelling and itching around the mouth and eyes, and she began vomiting and coughing. Her doctor treated the allergic reaction, and the woman had a satisfactory recovery.

Allergic reactions to psyllium are rare, but they can occur.

If you develop a strange allergic reaction after eating or handling psyllium, be sure to check with your doctor right away.

And if you are allergic to psyllium, be sure to read labels very carefully at the grocery store. Many high-fiber cereals and laxatives contain psyllium.

Colon Cancer

Antacid stops 75% of colon cancers?

Taking twice the current Recommended Dietary Allowance (RDA) of calcium every day might prevent nearly 75 percent of all colon cancers, says a cancer researcher in *Medical World News* (31,4:22).

That's equal to about eight regular non-prescription calcium carbonate antacid tablets.

Evidence of calcium's prevention power is snowballing, with 60 studies worldwide now reporting the mineral's natural benefits.

In light of these encouraging study results, some researchers are suggesting a change in the RDA of calcium for adults.

Currently, the RDA for people over 50 is 800 milligrams a day.

It takes 1,200 milligrams of calcium a day to prevent colon cancer in people under the age of 49, some pro-calcium researchers say.

People over age 49 need 1,500 milligrams daily to get the prevention effect, they suggest.

Check with your doctor before taking supplements of any kind, and especially before taking more than the RDA.

Colon cancer is the second deadliest cancer in the U.S, and each year, 145,000 new cases are diagnosed.

In 1987 alone, colon cancer killed 60,000 Americans.

Most of its victims are middle-aged or beyond.

The disease can be controlled and even cured if caught in its early stages.

Researchers really don't know how calcium works, but some believe it fights the effects of a high-fat diet on the colon wall, according to a report in *Preventive Medicine* (18,5:672).

Studies have shown that fatty foods speed up cell growth in the colon, and such spurts are the first step to tumor development.

Calcium travels throughout the digestive tract, working to keep cell growth under control.

It gets there by way of vitamin D — a rapid transit system of sorts — which transports energized calcium to the intestines, primed for preventing bad cell growth.

Although the experts agree that calcium does help fight colon cancer (and other diseases), they disagree on which form of calcium is best. Would a natural form of calcium be best?

Excellent natural sources of vitamin D are sunshine, tuna, fish liver oils and fortified milk.

You also can buy calcium supplements over-the-counter, meaning you don't need a doctor's prescription.

Taking eight carbonate tablets (such as Tums) a day would provide about 1,600 milligrams of calcium. (One regular Tums contains about 200 milligrams of calcium.)

If you take calcium supplements, you should drink at least two liters of fluid every day, recommends Dr. Cedric Garland, a professor at the University of California at San Diego.

Too much calcium and not enough fluids could add up to a case of painful kidney stones.

You shouldn't take more than 16 calcium carbonate tablets in a day nor for longer than two weeks.

Check with your doctor before taking antacids or any supplements.

Calcium has other benefits as well:

Heart disease. In one study, women who took 800 milligrams of calcium every day decreased their high blood pressure by 23 percent.

Women taking only 400 milligrams did not benefit as much.

High blood pressure is a serious heart-disease risk factor.

Bone disease. It's no secret that calcium promotes strong teeth and bones — but not just when you're young.

Dr. Robert P. Heany, of Creighton University in Omaha, Nebraska, notes the importance of calcium in two major stages of life:

(1) It helps develop bone mass during the first 30 years of life, and (2) then maintains bone mass during the remaining years of life.

However, as you get older, your body doesn't use calcium as efficiently as when you were young.

That's why you may need more calcium as you age, some researchers suggest.

Menopausal women may need even more calcium because their estrogen loss puts them at greater risk of developing osteoporosis.

For pregnant women, extra calcium may help prevent pre-eclampsia. This condition results in excessive fluid retention in the mother's body, which can kill the unborn child if not treated.

Salty diet linked to colorectal cancer

Australian researchers say people who eat an ounce or more

of salt a week face higher risks of getting colon and rectal cancers. The risk is greater for men than for women, says the report in *Nutrition and Cancer* (12,4:351). The same study also found that getting more potassium, particularly from fruits and vegetables, seems to protect men and women from both kinds of cancers.

Milk provides essential cancer-fighting elements

Mother was right when she told you to drink your milk. It could help save your life.

Just two eight-ounce glasses of fortified milk a day provide enough calcium and vitamin D to help lower your colon-cancer risk, according to *Medical World News* (31,1:41).

In a recent study, seven men at high risk for colon cancer took 1,250 milligrams of calcium every day for one week. In four men, extra calcium cut the amount of a cancer-causing enzyme in the colon by 50 percent.

This finding confirms several previous studies.

Researchers also found that people with higher levels of vitamin D — at least 20 milligrams per milliliter of blood serum — had a 70 percent decrease in colon-cancer risk compared to people with lower vitamin D levels (lower than 20 mg/ml).

So, drink your milk!

Sitting down to a steak dinner may be dangerous for your health

If you sit down to a meal of cheese steak very often, your colon may be paying a high, even deadly, price.

Those two actions — sitting a lot and consuming a lot of fatty meats and dairy products — are the very highest risk factors for developing colon and rectal cancers, says a major new study in the *Journal of the National Cancer Institute* (82,11:915).

The study of hundreds of Chinese in America and in China itself pointed at two main villains: saturated fat and a sedentary life-style.

In fact, the study found, your cancer risk increases as you spend more time sitting.

Eating more than 10 grams a day of saturated fat, along with physical inactivity, "could account for 60 percent of colon and rectal cancer incidence among Chinese-American men and 40 percent among Chinese-American women," the report says.

Ten grams is slightly more than one-third of one ounce.

Researchers compared the two groups because they wanted to find out why colon and rectal cancer rates are four to seven times higher among Chinese who move to America than rates among the general population in mainland China itself.

They took into account the difference in diets in the two countries.

For example, a typical mainland Chinese person will eat more calories per day than his Chinese-American cousin.

But more of those native-country calories will come from carbohydrates and starches.

In China, the average person will get about 54 percent of his protein requirements from grains like rice, and only 20 percent from meat (mainly pork) and fish, the report says.

Over here, however, the Chinese-American will reverse that — 60 percent of his protein from meat and fish, and only 17 percent from rice and other grains.

Both groups got about four to five grams a day of crude fiber.

Chinese-Americans took in more daily calcium and beta-carotene, a forerunner of vitamin A.

In this study, the two nutrients plus fiber seemed to give some protection against the two bowel cancers.

After accounting for diet differences, the two culprits of saturated fat and sedentary life-style stood out in the lineup as the major risk factors for developing colon and rectal cancer, this country's second-leading cancer killer.

Interestingly enough, people living in two mainland Chinese cities also had higher cancer rates, suggesting that city diets might not be as healthy as country diets.

Saturated fat is the stuff that makes butter and animal fat solid at room temperature.

Vegetable fats, on the other hand, usually contain monounsaturated and polyunsaturated fats and are generally liquid at room temperature.

Vegetable fats like corn oil and soybean oil make up most of the liquid cooking oils these days.

Nutritionists recommend that you eat foods low in saturated fats.

They suggest that you try to get less than a third of your daily calories from fats of all kinds, and less than one-tenth of your total calories from saturated fats.

Put the starch back into the diet

Years ago, starch was something other than what you spray on shirts to be ironed.

Starches were considered a distinct food group, and youngsters were encouraged to eat something from that group two or three times a day to ensure a healthy diet.

Come the Nineties, and starches are now "complex carbohydrates."

Despite the trendy name, starchy foods are still the same ones we knew as children: potatoes and rice and breads and foods made from grains.

One British researcher believes that starchy foods may be what's missing in our search for foods that protect from cancers of the colon and rectum.

No, it's not the fiber in those foods, either, although fiber certainly is beneficial.

Instead, believes K.W. Heaton of the Bristol Royal Infirmary in England, it's the starchy foods that "escape" digestion in the stomach and small intestine that may do us the most good.

Those "escaped" starches are quickly fermented in the large intestine (colon) and pass quickly on through the bowel.

The fermentation and quick passage seem to protect the colon from harmful substances in foods.

One clue supporting this theory is the finding that people who develop a lot of precancerous growths in their colons also seem to be unusually efficient at digesting starch before it gets to the colon, says Heaton.

Even those people could help themselves by eating starchy foods in less-digestible forms, the researcher suggests.

For example, instead of using baked flour products, eat a lot of whole grains like rice.

"Skin tags" provide clues for detecting colon cancer

Just about every second person over the age of 50 has skin tags.

These are little tumor stalks or flaps that protrude from the skin surface in the armpits, neck and groin area.

Usually skin tags cause no problems.

But, researchers are beginning to wonder whether the little stalks and flaps might be an early clue to tumors of the colon and rectum.

Colorectal tumors, of course, often turn into colon cancer.

Cancer of the colon or rectum is a slow-growing disease that will kill 60,000 people in the U.S.A. this year, reports Dr. J.R. Varma in *The Journal of the American Board of Family Practice* (3,3:175).

Colon cancer, caught in its early stages, is curable 90 percent of the time, the report says.

Those with skin tags were twice as likely as the general population to have tumorous growths, called polyps, in the colon, according to the article.

People under age 50 with skin tags were six times more likely to have colon polyps.

"Skin tags need to be considered a significant risk factor for polyps of the colon," says Dr. Varma. "I believe that [people] with large skin tags should be evaluated more closely."

That would include tests of bowel movements to look for hidden blood, X-rays using barium enemas and colonoscopy (viewing the inside of the colon through a tube).

Dietary fibers differ in fighting colorectal cancer

President Bush may not like broccoli, but your colon does!

According to *Nutrition and Cancer* (13,4:271), "vegetable fibers may generally be more protective against colorectal carcinogenesis (cancer) than cereals."

Vegetables are more "fermentable" than cereal fibers. Fermentation refers to the process in which the body (particularly the stomach and intestines) breaks down foods into usable compounds necessary for proper nutrition. A fiber source that is highly fermentable appears to be a strong warrior against cancer.

Fermentation takes place when the "good" bacteria in the intestines break down vegetable or animal matter. During that process, nutrients are released into the intestines. This process supplies the body with important nutrients. And, equally important, fermentation helps resupply the intestinal bacteria with vital nutrients. The bacteria help keep the bowel healthy and functioning properly and help protect the colon from cancer.

The *Nutrition and Cancer* report indicates that vegetable and cereal fibers release a continuous stream of nutrients, unlike some starches and sugars. Carbohydrates from starches and sugars break down rapidly and might actually increase the risk of colorectal cancer.

With a garden of varieties to choose from, vegetables sprout up as a healthy alternative for your fight against colon cancer.

Common bean and pea help reduce the risk of cancer

It's no longer a secret — the food on your dinner plate can greatly influence your health. In fact, if you choose your menu wisely, you can actually build a line of defense against cancer.

The common bean and pea are two kinds of those cancer-fighting foods, reports *Nutrition and Cancer* (14,2:85). In a recent study, those people who frequently ate legumes (beans, peas, lentils, soybeans, etc.) cut their risk of colon and rectal cancer in half.

The secret behind the anti-cancer effects of legumes is a substance known as protease inhibitor (PI). Protease inhibitor is a strong anti-cancer ingredient, and legumes contain high concentrations of this cancer-fighting substance.

Another plus: adding more foods with a high PI content to your diet helps protect you from colon and rectal cancer without

Diabetes

Check your feet for blood sugar disorders

The ulcer that recently has developed on your foot may be a blessing in disguise. It could be the tell-tale sign that your doctor needs to diagnose a blood-sugar disorder that has gone undetected for years.

According to a report in the *British Medical Journal* (300,6731:1046), about 15 percent of all diabetic people develop foot ulcers, and most foot ulcers are directly associated with diabetes. So, if you develop a foot ulcer, you have a strong chance of having diabetes.

Some studies have indicated that foot ulcers may be associated with smoking, although many scientists doubt this theory. Foot ulcers have also been linked with other disorders such as vascular disease (blood vessel disease).

Because a foot ulcer could have various causes or even several causes, it is important for you to have it evaluated right away to avoid further complications.

Researchers recommend that if you develop a foot ulcer, you should check with your doctor immediately for a diabetes test and possibly go to a special diabetic service for a full evaluation.

Pass the pasta to conserve chromium and avoid diabetes

The spaghetti you eat today may help keep you healthy tomorrow! Researchers now believe that eating a diet that conserves the mineral chromium may prevent the development of a form of diabetes called Type II diabetes.

This form of diabetes usually affects adults over forty who are overweight. The people who risk developing this non-insulin-dependent form of diabetes are not able to absorb the blood sugar (glucose) from their bloodstreams properly and are said to be "glucose intolerant."

Your doctor can give you a simple test that will reveal whether you have mild glucose intolerance, the condition that precedes Type II diabetes. If you are mildly glucose-intolerant, don't worry! You may still be able to avoid diabetes with certain changes in your diet.

The key is to increase the amount of chromium in your body. According to *Science News* (137,14:214), chromium can improve your ability to use blood sugar and help prevent the development of Type II diabetes.

Unfortunately, it's not that easy to increase your chromium. You can eat high-chromium foods like meat, cheese, whole-grain breads and cereals, broccoli, potatoes, and some fruits, wines and beers. But your body can't easily absorb the chromium from all these natural sources.

Researchers suggest another approach to try in combination with a chromium-rich diet: stay away from foods rich in simple sugars such as fructose and glucose. These foods cause your body to excrete large amounts of chromium.

On the other hand, eating foods that are high in complex carbohydrates, such as pasta, will help you conserve the chromium in your body.

Ask your doctor's advice. If you have mild glucose intolerance, or even if you have already developed Type II diabetes, you may be able to improve your glucose tolerance just by changing your diet.

Magnesium helps lower blood pressure in Type II diabetes

You've heard the old saying that "an apple a day keeps the doctor away."

The next verse could go something like this: "A fresh salad a day helps keep hypertension away."

It seems that eating a fresh green salad with lunch every day may help lower your blood pressure if you suffer from high blood pressure and Type II diabetes.

What's so great about a green salad? you ask.

Green, leafy vegetables found in fresh salads are good sources of the mineral magnesium. Magnesium is an important mineral in the human body, and studies show that a magnesium deficiency may contribute to high blood pressure, reports the Sept. 22, 1990 *Science News* (138,12:189).

Eating green vegetables every day helps increase the amount of magnesium in the body. And a magnesium-enriched diet may help lower high blood pressure by relaxing constricted (tightened) blood vessels.

Recent studies suggest that people with high blood pressure and Type II diabetes have low levels of magnesium in their red blood cells.

So, researchers think that many Type II diabetics could help control their high blood pressure by taking magnesium supplements or by eating foods rich in magnesium.

However, they warn that magnesium supplements could be dangerous for some diabetics.

Apparently, some people with diabetes can experience kidney problems that could result in dangerously high levels of magnesium in the blood. Therefore, researchers recommend that all diabetic people consult their doctors before taking any magnesium supplements.

New sweetener safe and ideal for diabetics

Diabetics and dieters! Have you ever wanted a sweetener that is safe, sweet and tasty? Well, thanks to some Danish scientist, you may soon have one, claims *The American Journal of Clinical Nutrition* (52,4:675).

The Jerusalem artichoke can provide a kind of natural sugar called fructan that might fulfill all of your requirements for a sweetener.

This new sweetener has two main benefits:

1. Low in calories. Fructan has long molecules instead of the short molecules found in most common sugars. Your body cannot absorb the long fructan molecules very well. This means that you may take in a lot of calories by using the sweetener, but you won't have to suffer the consequences because your body can't "use" the sugar.

2. Stabilizes blood sugar levels. Fructan does not appear to cause a drastic change in blood sugar levels.

Eating carbohydrates usually raises blood glucose levels.

But, when fructan is used, the blood sugar levels appear to be lowered instead of raised.

And fructan seems to reduce the body's need for insulin, which is great news for diabetics!

Scientists are still researching and studying fructan, but some forms of fructan are already on the market.

If you are on a special diet or are taking insulin or other medicines, check with your doctor before using fructan products.

Digestive Disorders

Do you abuse laxatives?

Do you have diarrhea, cramping, nausea and vomiting, but your doctor can't find anything wrong with you?

If you use laxatives, you may be overdoing it, says a report in *Medical World News* (31,1:19).

Regularity doesn't necessarily mean daily bowel movements, the article points out. Many people don't realize the dangers associated with laxatives and thus use them much too often.

Laxative abuse is commonly defined as using a laxative at least once a week over a period of several months, according to the report.

"Patients risk nutritional deficiencies, metabolic disorders, and potentially severe damage to the gastrointestinal tract with regular, long-term use of laxatives," according to experts at an American College of Gastroenterology meeting.

Over-the-counter laxative abuse is very hard to diagnose because the symptoms are similar to those of other common intestinal disorders. And doctors often fail to ask about laxatives when questioning patients about medication use.

If you think you are overusing laxatives, experts suggest that you eat more foods high in dietary fiber, drink more fluids and begin a progressive exercise program.

That combination will give you the same results as the laxatives without the harmful side effects of laxative overuse.

Bananas for indigestion pain?

Bothered by indigestion pain? Eat a banana!

That's the essence of a study by researchers in India, reports *The Lancet* (335,8689:612).

They took 40 people — each of whom had experienced many months of stomach pain and nausea but who had no ulcers — and tried a natural remedy on half of them.

The researchers gave 20 of them capsules containing banana powder — eight capsules a day for eight weeks. The second group of 20 took nothing for the discomfort. All of them stayed away from antacids or ulcer medicines.

By study's end, half of those who took banana pills reported complete relief, and another one-fourth received at least some relief from their constant indigestion problems.

In the other group, eight out of 10 still had indigestion problems.

Bananas are a common food in India, and many Indians also use banana powder, a dried and ground-up form of the fruit, the report says.

Banana powder also protects the stomach lining from irritation by aspirin and some other drugs, say the report authors, and has been used with some success in treating ulcer symptoms. No side effects were reported.

Try iced tea instead

Hot drinks, such as tea and coffee, can give you an ulcer, British researchers report in *Gut* (30:1201, 1989)

The hotter the drink, the more damage done to the protective lining of the stomach.

The lining protects the stomach from acid attack.

Fight the "flu" — loosen up

Your flu-like illness might not be caused by germs.

You simply may be wearing your seat belt shoulder strap too tight.

A tight belt can rub against your neck and irritate the thyroid gland. This is known as thyroiditis and can cause fever, neck pain and a flu-like illness, reports a digest in *Bottom Line* (9,13:4).

Simple treatment: loosen your seat belt just a little.

If your flu-like symptoms don't disappear, check with your doctor. You might have the real flu!

Spice for life

Ginger is believed by some to be one of the better natural stomach "medicines" around.

Ginger seems to help prevent stomach ulcers, says a digest in *HerbalGram* (20:23).

It also is used commonly to prevent or calm motion sickness, morning sickness, or just general nausea.

Get your head up

If your sleep has been constantly interrupted by problems with heartburn, try elevating the head of your bed.

Researchers in England have found that a 9-inch "lift" to the head of the bed provides great relief for nighttime heartburn, says a report in *The Lancet* (2,8569:1200).

Relief from diarrhea

The most important thing you can do if you're suffering from diarrhea is to replace the fluids your body is losing, says a report in *Medical Abstracts* (10,2:2). Even if you're nauseated and sick at your stomach, you need to try to force some liquids down.

Try to take frequent small sips of liquids such as Gatorade, fruit drinks, chicken broth without fat, and non-diet non-caffeinated soft drinks.

Try to drink at least two quarts of liquids a day. And drink three quarts if you have a fever, the report suggests.

Can 'harmless' heartburn harm your heart?

■ Heart—For years, doctors have warned us not to mistake the warning symptoms of a heart attack for what they considered "harmless" heartburn.

Now, new studies suggest that heartburn itself might represent a real threat to your heart's health.

That burning or gnawing pain below the breastbone is triggered when stomach acid backs up into your esophagus, the food tube between the mouth and stomach.

We call it heartburn. Doctors call it gastroesophageal reflux.

A University of Maryland doctor reports that such acid back-ups actually can slow down the heartbeat by 20 beats a minute in otherwise healthy people.

Slowing down the heart rate could be dangerous for people with heart disease and previous heart attacks, says the report in *Geriatrics* (45,7:22).

Because of the risk involved with a slowed-down heart, doctors should be "aggressive" in treating reflux, especially among the elderly and people with heart-rhythm problems, says the report.

If you have heart disease and suffer regular episodes of heartburn, ask your doctor about this report in the July 1990 edition of *Geriatrics*.

■ Lungs — That acid back-up into the esophagus might also trigger unexplained coughing and even asthma, says an editorial in *The Lancet* (336,8710:282).

About one out of every 10 chronic coughers could get relief by getting treatment for acid reflux, or heartburn, the article suggests.

A super-fine acid spray from the stomach possibly irritates lung and esophagus tissues, causing wheezing and asthmatic breathing spasms, the editorial says.

Some natural heartburn remedies include the following:

* Taking banana powder
* Raising the head of your bed by six to eight inches
* Avoiding food or drink for at least two hours before bedtime
* Losing weight, especially around the middle
* Sucking on candy-like lozenges (except peppermint-flavored ones)
* Eating more slowly, according to *New Natural Healing Encyclopedia* (FC&A, 1990: pg.193)

Check with your doctor about heartburn treatments.

Treatment helps heal 9 out of 10 peptic ulcers

You know the symptoms. The burning, gnawing and aching feeling in your stomach means your peptic ulcer has flared up — again.

The antacids relieve the pain and discomfort for a while, but you can't seem to find any long-term relief. And your doctor can't seem to find a cure.

Until now, that is.

Scientists may have found a way to prevent ulcers from flaring up in people who have histories of recurring peptic ulcers, reports the October 1990 *Medical World News* (31,16:17).

Scientists now think that peptic ulcers might be linked to a kind of bacteria known as *Helicobacter pylori*. The scientists' theory is that if they can eliminate the bacteria, they can eliminate the ulcers.

And their research seems to support this theory.

Until recently, doctors have enjoyed only temporary success in the treatment of ulcers. More than 80 percent of all ulcers that were treated reappeared after the treatment ended. As a result, those with ulcers had to take continuous doses of medicine to prevent the ulcers from reappearing.

However, scientists now believe that the *H. pylori* bacterium is the key to ending this frustrating cycle. So, they have been focusing on a treatment that kills the bacteria.

The researchers found that killing the bacteria resulted in zero cases of peptic ulcer relapse at the end of one year. In other words, killing and removing the bacteria "cured" the ulcer and prevented it from recurring.

Studies show that nine out of 10 people who suffer from ulcer flare-ups have *H. pylori* bacteria present in their digestive tract. So researchers think that killing the bacteria would eliminate ulcer flare-ups in nine out of 10 people suffering from ulcer disease.

One of the drugs used to eliminate the bacteria and prevent the ulcer from recurring is not currently available for doctors to use. However, doctors and researchers remain excited about the possibilities of eliminating the plague of peptic ulcers.

Drug and Food Reactions

Commonly prescribed sedatives contribute to falling accidents

The medicine in the most commonly prescribed sedative may play a major role in causing older people to fall, leading to more broken hips, says a study in *The Journal of the American Medical Association* (262,23:3303).

The tranquilizer ingredient is benzodiazepine. It or closely related drugs are found in Valium, Xanax, Tranxene, Ativan, Serax, Centrax, Paxipam, Librium and Libritabs, Limbitrol and Menrium brands.

In the study, people over 65 who used the long-acting benzodiazepine faced a risk of broken hip nearly double that of people who took other kinds of tranquilizers, according to the *JAMA* report.

"For older patients, a serious consequence of [using]...benzodiazepines may be an increased risk of falling and fall-related fractures," say the researchers.

They recommend that doctors avoid prescribing this kind of tranquilizer and sleeping pill for people over 65, the report says.

If you are taking this medication, talk with your doctor before changing or discontinuing use of the drug.

Side effects of antidepressants could be hazardous to your health

If your doctor has prescribed medication to ease depression, take note: some antidepressants may do more harm than good if you have a heart condition.

This warning comes from researchers at the Mayo Clinic in Rochester, Minn., who say doctors should fully evaluate a person's health before prescribing an antidepressant.

The most common side effect of antidepressants is low blood pressure, which in the elderly may lead to stroke and heart attack and sometimes results in death.

Side effects may be more harmful in the elderly because they often take many different medications, which may interact with one another.

Elderly people are also more sensitive to certain drugs, so dosage is important.

Here's a look at a few common antidepressants and their side effects:

Imipramine: Low blood pressure, erratic heart rhythm, increased heart rate, heart block (the heart works at less than capacity).

Maprotiline: Heart block, low blood pressure, nerve disorders, seizures.

Trazodone: Low blood pressure, irregular heart beat.

Perhaps the safest antidepressant for the heart is **fluoxetine**. Although studies have shown that it slightly decreases the resting heart rate, it has caused very few, if any, heart problems.

Generally, antidepressants are safe and effective. If you take an antidepressant and have had side effects, or are concerned about them, talk to your doctor.

Treatment for one form of cancer may cause another kind of cancer

Women who undergo chemotherapy for ovarian cancer have a higher risk than usual of developing leukemia later on, according to a report in *The New England Journal of Medicine* (322,1:1).

Studies in Europe, England and Canada have identified several factors that work together to increase a woman's leukemia risk:

• **Age.** The older a woman is at the time of cancer diagnosis, the higher her leukemia risk. During the studies, at the time of diagnosis, at least half the women were 58 or older.

• **Stage of cancer.** Women in an advanced stage of ovarian cancer are more likely to get leukemia after chemotherapy because they need more chemicals to fight advanced cancer. An early cancer diagnosis cuts the leukemia risk, the report says.

• **Type of treatment.** Women with ovarian cancer who are treated with surgery alone have the least chance of developing leukemia later on. Those who are treated with radiotherapy have a slightly higher risk.

Chemotherapy alone presents the highest risk, researchers say. The risk of radiotherapy and chemotherapy combined is a bit lower, possibly because smaller doses of chemotherapy drugs are used.

• **Type of chemotherapy drug used.** During the study, researchers identified five chemotherapy drugs that increase the leukemia risk: chlorambucil, cyclophosphamide, melphalan, thiotepa and treosulfan.

The risk depends on dosage and whether the drugs are used

in combination — the current trend in ovarian cancer treatment, researchers say.

• **Time elapsed after chemotherapy.** Women are more likely to get leukemia four to six years after beginning chemotherapy (or one to four years after finishing it), although the risk is still significant even 10 years later.

Researchers point out that chemotherapy is becoming a popular treatment for women with ovarian cancer.

At this point, they aren't sure whether the benefits outweigh the leukemia risks, the report says.

There are no set rules or guidelines about cancer-therapy risks. Each woman is treated individually.

If you have ovarian cancer, ask your doctor to fully explain the risks and side effects of each form of treatment.

Be persistent. You need all of the facts before you and your family can choose the therapy that will give you the greatest benefit with the lowest risk.

Glaucoma eyedrops may react with other prescribed medications

Are you suffering from light-headedness, nausea, vomiting, memory loss, blurry vision and fatigue, and your doctor doesn't know why?

If you have glaucoma, your eyedrops could be the culprit, according to a report in the *Annals of Internal Medicine* (112,2:120).

Headache, tremors, disorientation, bowel distress, and lower heart rate and blood pressure are just some of the side effects that have been linked with glaucoma medications.

If you have any of these side effects accompanying your eye problems, see your doctor right away.

Most people with glaucoma are elderly, and they may be taking other medications to treat a host of medical problems.

Although most glaucoma medications are made to reduce pressure in the eye itself, various amounts of the drug can be absorbed through the tear ducts, interacting with other medications in the body.

Gentle pressure on the tear ducts can help reduce the amount of glaucoma drug absorbed by your body.

Experts recommend that you lie down while putting in eyedrops and apply only one drop at a time.

After putting in eyedrops, hold a soft tissue to your tear ducts in the inside corners of your eyes for five minutes.

But the best thing you can do to prevent drug side effects is to let all your doctors know what medications you take. That includes over-the-counter medicines and even vitamin and mineral supplements.

Your eye doctor and family physician probably don't talk with each other about your health and about the medications you're taking, so it's up to you to keep them informed.

Heart medication caution

A type of drug commonly prescribed to control heart problems may cause a persistent, dry cough in some people warns a report in *Emergency Medicine* (22,4:8).

The culprits: angiotensin-converting enzyme inhibitors (a.k.a. ACE inhibitors), which help improve blood flow.

If you take an ACE inhibitor and have these symptoms without sore throat or fever, see your doctor.

Is microwaved food safe to eat?

Fluffy popcorn, crispy-crust pizza, and crunchy fried chicken in just minutes.

The microwave is surely one of the greatest conveniences of all time, but recently consumer groups have raised questions about the safety of microwave packaging — those plastic trays, wraps and bags that magically brown and crisp foods.

According to the *Nutrition Action Health Letter* (17,1:5), "microwave ovens can't brown and crisp foods on their own."

The "magic" is heat-susceptor packaging, which acts as a "little frying pan," says Food and Drug Administration chemist Les Borodinsky.

That little frying pan is actually thin, gray strips of polyethylene terpthalate (PET) on the bottom of the package. (You can sometimes see the strips if you hold the package up to the light.)

The FDA says PET is safe to use at 300 degrees F, but when PET reaches higher temperatures, it breaks down and releases chemicals into food. In the microwave, PET can reach 500 degrees or higher.

According to the *Health Letter*, heat-susceptor packages often contain a number of chemicals — "all known or suspected carcinogens" — that can be released into the foods. Carcinogens are cancer-causing agents.

Some of the chemicals are not actually part of PET, but rather are part of the adhesive strips that hold PET on the package.

No one really knows which types of containers are microwave-safe. According to the *Health Letter*, the FDA doesn't regulate trays, containers and plastic wraps used in microwave cooking at home.

Although a manufacturer may claim its containers are microwave-safe, no FDA safety standards exist, so you really can't be sure whether the product is in fact safe.

Until the FDA begins to regulate microwave-safe packaging, the *Health Letter* offers these tips to keep your family safe:

■ Avoid frozen "pizza, french fries, waffles, popcorn, breaded fish, and other food that use heat-susceptor packaging."

■ Some foods are packaged so that you can cook them in a microwave or conventional oven (the package will have directions for both cooking methods). This type of packaging doesn't contain heat-susceptors but still releases chemicals into food, even when heated in a conventional oven.

To avoid this hazard, transfer all such foods from the plastic trays to glass cookware, which is the safest type container to use in the microwave. (At this point, Corning Ware appears safe.)

■ Don't cover glass containers with plastic. The chemicals that give plastic wraps their "cling" could poison your food if overheated in the microwave. Use glass covers, or, if you must use plastic wrap, don't let it touch the food.

■ Don't use margarine tubs to reheat leftovers. They'll eventually melt and release chemicals into your food.

Stressed out? Put down that coffee cup

If you have a high-stress job, put down your coffee cup.

University of Oklahoma researchers say more than five cups of coffee a day can send your blood pressure soaring, reports *Modern Medicine* (57,11:22).

Thirty-four men took a simple test. They drank two glasses

of grapefruit juice, one containing the amount of caffeine equal to that in two or three cups of coffee.

Their blood pressures were measured 15 minutes after finishing each glass.

Before the test, 17 men were identified at high risk for hypertension, the medical name for high blood pressure.

Risk factors include diet and a parent with high blood pressure.

After drinking the caffeinated juice, their blood pressures were higher than the low-risk men.

Although coffee has not been proven to increase the risk of heart disease, another team of researchers recommends that people with heart problems drink decaffeinated coffee or no coffee at all, says another report in *Modern Medicine* (57,11:118).

Driving under the influence of ... antihistamines?

Taking a common, over-the-counter antihistamine might affect you in the same way as drinking several quick shots of liquor, two independent studies suggest.

The kinds of antihistamines that cause sleepiness also can knock precious seconds off your reaction time while driving an automobile, says a report in *Medical World News* (31,11:19).

In one test, two hours after taking a pill containing diphenhydramine, men reacted to traffic hazards half as quickly as when they took a fake pill.

Their slowed reactions were about the same as drivers with 0.10 percent blood alcohol level. A driver with that level of blood alcohol is considered legally drunk in most states.

Diphenhydramine also is the active ingredient in several nonprescription sleeping pills.

Another test used the antihistamine triprolidine. Driver impairment was equivalent to a drinking driver with 0.06 percent blood alcohol, enough to get you in trouble with the law in many states.

Although most over-the-counter antihistamines contain package warnings against driving while using the nonprescription medicines, more than six out of 10 people ignore the instructions, the report says.

Since people vary in their responses even to so-called sedative-type antihistamines, a blanket prohibition against driving after taking a sneezing-sniffling pill probably is "inappropriate," the report concludes.

Several newer types of antihistamines don't cause sleepiness. Tests of the newer, non-sedating medicines also don't show any driving impairment, the report says.

Products containing sedative-type antihistamines

The following products contain sleep-inducing antihistamines:

- Diphenhydramine
- Alka-Seltzer Plus Night-Time Cold Medicine
- Excedrin PM tablets and caplets
- Benadryl syrup, tablets, spray and capsules
- Demarest
- Miles Nervine Nighttime Sleep-Aid
- Nytol tablets
- Sleep-eze 3 tablets
- Sleepinal Night-time Sleep Aid capsules
- Sominex tablets and liquid
- Sominex Pain Relief formula

- Unisom Dual Relief Nighttime Sleep Aid/Analgesic
- Triprolidine
- Actidil syrup and tablets
- Actifed capsules, syrup and tablets
- Actifed Plus caplets and tablets
- Actifed 12-Hour capsules
- AllerAct caplets and tablets

Source: *Physicians Desk Reference for Nonprescription Drugs,* 1990 Edition

---

Flying high or nose dive — it's all in the medication

One common medicine for high blood pressure seems to cause a nose dive in people's quality of life, while another kind seems to give people a nice boost, reports an *Associated Press* story.

People taking the prescription beta blocker propranolol reported that it seemed to worsen their sex lives, emotions, work and sleep habits.

But people taking the calcium channel blocker nicardipine said they noticed improvements in all those areas.

Both classes of drugs work about equally well in controlling high blood pressure, says Dr. Lars G. Ekelund.

He talked about the study at the 13th meeting of the International Society of Hypertension in Montreal in June 1990.

Another strike against beta blockers: this class of drug increases LDL ("bad") cholesterol and lowers HDL, the "good" form.

That raises people's risk of heart disease, the report says.

112

Name brand or generic — there's more at stake than cost alone

Many pharmacists routinely give consumers the generic brand of a drug rather than the prescribed "name brand" because the generic brand is usually less expensive.

However, the few pennies you save might not be worth the trouble you might get in return.

Some researchers believe that some generic substitute drugs are not as effective as the matching prescribed brand-name drugs and could even cause severe problems.

The Journal of the American Medical Association (263,18:2459) reports a recent case in which a 28-year-old man had been taking a drug to help his pancreas function correctly. He had been taking the drug for approximately 25 years with no reported side effects or problems.

One month, his pharmacist replaced the prescribed drug with a generic brand of that drug, and the man immediately began having problems.

He telephoned his doctor about the problems that had developed, and his doctor changed the drug back to the original kind.

The man's negative side effects disappeared within one week, and he had no more complaints thereafter.

Usually, generic drugs perform exactly as the prescribed medications do, and consumers have no problems with negative side effects.

However, if you suddenly develop unexplained side effects after switching to a generic drug, ask your doctor or pharmacist to determine if the generic drug is causing the problem.

Careful, though — don't stop taking your medicine without checking with your doctor first.

"Take only as directed..."

How closely you follow the directions on your medicine bottles will determine how effective your medicines will be.

Food can either help or hurt the effectiveness of the medications.

So, medications that should be taken with food are obviously most effective when taken with food.

When taken on an empty stomach, the medications don't work as well.

And medications that should not be taken with food lose some of their effectiveness if taken on a full stomach, reports *The Lancet* (335, 8689:597).

If you have questions about when or how to take your medicine, be sure to contact your doctor or pharmacist immediately.

It could make the difference between sickness and health for you.

Check the scale, then check the medicine cabinet

Before you start blaming yourself for an unexpected weight gain, maybe you should check your medicine cabinet.

A study reported in the *British Medical Journal* (300,6729:902) suggests that weight gain may be a side effect of long-term use of propranolol, a beta-blocker used for heart problems.

According to *BMJ*, the medicinal weight gain was seen in both men and women involved in a 40-month study, and the weight gain wasn't limited to any age group.

Although the weight increase was moderate, it was in addition to any other weight differences due to aging or overeating.

Because some people suffer physically or emotionally from even a slight increase in weight, the news that medication can cause a further gain is important.

Weight gain is never a simple problem.

Why one person can eat anything and remain thin, while another person counts calories and still gains has always been difficult to answer.

Obviously metabolism plays an important part, but to further complicate the matter, certain medications bring about undeserved gain.

These pounds seem especially hard to control since eating and exercise habits aren't to blame.

Your doctor will advise you if it's important to your health to take propranolol.

Always follow his advice — just be aware that a gradual increase in weight may accompany the medical benefits of the drug.

Blood pressure drugs may trigger diabetes cases

Diabetes in middle-aged men may be brought on by treatment with prescription drugs used to lower high blood pressure, according to a new report in the *British Medical Journal* (298,6681:1147).

Men treated for high blood pressure were more likely to develop diabetes than men with normal blood pressure who were not taking medication, says Dr. Einar T. Skarfors, leader of the nine-year study in Sweden.

Treatment with blood pressure drugs seemed to be most harmful in men who were "predisposed" to diabetes, Skarfors explained.

Men with high risk factors for diabetes, like an immediate relative with diabetes, a low insulin index or extremely high blood pressure, were most likely to develop diabetes while on blood pressure reducing drugs.

The study focused on the second number in a blood pressure reading, known as the diastolic pressure. It measures the pressure of blood in the arteries while the heart rests between beats.

According to the *Journal*, "the incidence of diabetes was seven times higher among men whose diastolic blood pressure had been greater than 105 mm Hg than among those in whom it had been less than 85 mm Hg."

A diastolic level of less than 85 mm Hg is considered normal. But a reading of more than 105 is considered high and a potential health risk.

Today's most commonly prescribed blood pressure drugs "may cause a decrease in insulin sensitivity which does not disappear with time," according to the report.

Continued use of these blood pressure-reducing drugs may actually trigger diabetes, the report says.

The study "does not prove" that this drug therapy causes some cases of diabetes.

But it does support the theory that long-term treatment with blood pressure reducing drugs may increase the chance of developing diabetes, Skarfors writes.

The prescription drugs taken by the men in the study were propranolol, hydralazine, atenolol, metoprolol and thiazide diuretics (also known as water pills).

Anti-arrhythmic drug side effects may defeat the purpose of the drug

Could the heart medication you've been taking to prevent

dangerous irregular heartbeats actually be **creating** irregular heartbeats and increasing your risk of sudden death? Many researchers think so.

According to a recent news release from the American Heart Association (March 1990:1), "anti-arrhythmic drugs, rather than protecting against life-threatening irregular heartbeats, may actually worsen some patient's conditions and possibly increase the risk of sudden death."

Apparently, anti-arrhythmic drugs prevent one kind of life-threatening irregular heartbeat (arrhythmia), but they also **cause** a different kind of irregular heartbeat that may cause sudden death.

Most doctors prescribe anti-arrhythmic drugs for people with congestive heart failure in an effort to cut the high death rate among these patients.

This practice could be changing now. "A lot of people are taking anti-arrhythmic drugs who don't need them," says Dr. Milton Packer in the March issue of *Circulation*, an American Heart Association journal.

Doctors are beginning to think that this drug therapy should be limited to patients with serious arrhythmias that cause significant symptoms or are life-threatening. In these serious cases, the benefits of the drug may outweigh the risks.

If you are taking anti-arrhythmic drugs, you may want to ask your doctor to reevaluate their need in light of the new studies. But do not stop taking these medications on your own.

Stopping the drug therapy without checking with your doctor could be just as dangerous.

Ibuprofen: friend or foe?

Millions of Americans rely on non-prescription pain killers

to help with arthritis pain and other on-going physical problems. The group of medicines most often recommended fall in the category of nonsteroidal anti-inflammatory drug (NSAID) therapy.

Ibuprofen heads the list in effectiveness and widespread use, but according to a study conducted at the Johns Hopkins University School of Medicine, it isn't a panacea.

The Annals of Internal Medicine (112,8:568) reports findings of this study, which was created to learn more about the effects of NSAIDs on the kidneys. A group of twelve women, ranging in ages from 28 to 75 years, were given 800 milligrams of ibuprofen three times daily for eleven days.

Their renal function was then closely monitored for signs of renal failure. Kidney function in these women was considered "stable" if adequate amounts of prostaglandins, an ingredient necessary for the regulation of healthy renal activity, was found to be present at normal levels. Prostaglandins play a critical role in people over 60 years old, or in anyone with circulatory problems, such as kidney failure or liver disease.

When, through urine analysis, ibuprofen was found to suppress the prostaglandin levels below those considered healthy, its use was discontinued. It was at this level where ibuprofen-induced, severe renal failure occurred.

In most cases, renal failure brought on by ibuprofen is reversible once the constant doses are discontinued.

But the message here seems to suggest moderation in your intake before a problem can occur.

Remember to work closely with your doctor, especially if you suspect any change in the way your pain-reliever is effecting your general health.

Recurrent NSAID use can result in GI complications or even death

The aspirin you've been taking for your headache may be causing your stomachache!

Aspirin is in the class of drugs known as nonsteroidal anti-inflammatory drugs (NSAIDs). These drugs are easily obtained and in wide use as non-prescription pain killers, but studies are beginning to suggest that regular use of these common medications may be more dangerous than previously believed.

Researchers from both the United States and England have verified that serious internal bleeding problems often are associated with NSAIDs. *Geriatrics* (45,4:18) reports in a recent study that more than one-third of all hospital admissions for bleeding ulcers in British hospitals were directly linked to these drugs — especially in persons over age 60.

Dr. James F. Fries, Associate Professor of Medicine at Stanford University Medical Center in California, warns that all people who have experienced previous upper abdominal pain and anyone taking antacids or certain digestive medications are probably in a high risk category for GI (gastrointestinal) disturbances. Smokers and persons taking corticosteroids also need to be alert to signs of GI disturbances.

Check with your doctor or pharmacist about the pros and cons of the medications you take regularly. A doctor familiar with your health needs can help you determine whether the use of NSAIDs is best for you.

Photocopy blues

If you've been suffering from hay-fever symptoms, but none of your hay-fever remedies have worked, you may be reacting to the Xerox machine in your office building or local drug store.

A recent report in *The New England Journal of Medicine* (322,18:1323) states that nasal stuffiness, headaches, and other common allergy-like reactions may be caused by laser printers and photocopying machines.

Apparently, the machines give off emissions which contain some volatile organic compounds that have been associated with this allergic reaction.

Inadequate air circulation inside the buildings that house laser printers and photocopying machines leads to "stale" air that contains these emissions and results in headaches, sore throats and runny noses, often referred to as "sick building syndrome."

If you suspect you're suffering from "sick building syndrome," you may consider spending as little time around these culprit machines as possible.

Occasional breaths of fresh air away from the machines may be all you need to clear up your symptoms.

Be sure to check with your doctor if you have questions about this condition.

Beware of mixing drugs

If you take a number of medications and suffer from agitation, confusion, delirium and dry mouth, you may be overdosing yourself, according to *Drug Therapy* (19,11:45).

For example, if you take three medications — two prescription and one over-the-counter — that happen to produce the same side effects, the side effects will be tripled.

Always tell your doctor about *every* medication you take, and ask your pharmacist whether prescription drugs can be used with over-the-counter drugs.

And store them safely

The Food and Drug Administration recommends storing your medications in a cool, dry place — not the bathroom.

One drug in particular, carbamazepine (brand name Tegretol), which is taken to prevent epileptic seizures, can "lose one-third of its effectiveness if it is stored in humid conditions," such as a bathroom, the FDA says.

Poor storage may explain why some epileptic patients complain that carbamazepine sometimes doesn't work for them.

Don't cool your drugs!

Store all drugs and medications at room temperature unless otherwise directed by your doctor or pharmacist.

Refrigerating drugs can change the way they work, endangering your health, says a digest in *Bottom Line* (9,13:4).

Ask your doctor or pharmacist if it's safe to put your medication in the "fridge."

Microwaving may contribute to food poisoning

British researchers believe they may have found a hidden danger in microwaving prepared foods. The amount of salt or sugar in these foods may change the way the foods absorb microwave energy, says a report in *Science News* (137,14:215).

Researchers found that a high salt or sugar content prevents foods from reaching a high enough temperature to kill salmonella and other dangerous bacteria. In fact, microwaving may only heat these bacteria to a temperature that helps them grow rather than kills them.

To avoid food poisoning, researchers agree that you should microwave foods longer and at a lower temperature than the package recommends. Then let the food sit for a few minutes to make sure dangerous bacteria have been killed.

Feeling dizzy and disoriented?

If you've been feeling dizzy and fuzzy lately, too much aspirin may be the culprit! According to research just published in *Geriatrics (45,4:20)*, taking aspirin regularly can actually cause a form of intoxication in some older people known as salicylism. This may occur even if you are taking the proper dosage of aspirin!

Older people may be more likely to react to aspirin because of smaller body mass, side effects from other drugs taken at the same time, or from a slower metabolism. But the good news is that researchers have found that this problem improves when people stop taking aspirin.

Arthritis drugs cause severe kidney damage

Commonly prescribed arthritis medicines known as NSAIDs cause reversible kidney failure in some elderly people, reports Dr. Jerry H. Gurwitz in the July 25, 1990 *The Journal of the American Medical Association* (264,4:471).

The nonsteroidal anti-inflammatory drugs fight pain and inflammation in arthritis conditions.

But people in their seventies, eighties and nineties seem to face increased chances of developing a condition called azotemia from high doses.

In azotemia, the kidneys falter and unhealthy levels of nitrogen waste products like urea get into the bloodstream.

Take away the high doses of NSAIDs, says the article, and most people get better within two weeks.

However, you should always check with your doctor before you stop taking medications.

Anti-baldness drug can cause pain and burning

Four men tried a prescription hair grower, minoxidil, to fight their baldness.

In addition to hair, though, they got severe cases of pain and burning sensations in the shoulders, pelvic girdle, arms and legs, reports a letter to the editor in the Aug.1 1990 issue of *Annals of Internal Medicine* (113,3:256).

Minoxidil was the only medicine they were taking. They applied it to their scalps twice a week for two to 14 months.

In addition to the days and nights of severe pain (called polymyalgia), some of them suffered loss of taste, loss of appetite, weight loss, chest pains and fatigue.

Doctors took them off the hair-growing medicine, and all their symptoms disappeared, the report says.

When eating vegetables can be dangerous

"Eat your veggies!" may be very bad advice for a few people.

In fact, for a small group of people, eating vegetables regularly could literally shorten their lives!

These few are people with a rare genetic disorder called phytosterolemia.

This condition causes a person to absorb a large amount of plant sterols (vegetable fats) from regular vegetables.

Someone with phytosterolemia has a high level of sterols in the blood and increased numbers of fatty deposits under the skin, resulting in little tumor-like growths on the eyelids, buttocks and other places.

Such a person also has a higher risk of developing hardened arteries and blocked blood vessels, says an article in *Diet and Health* (pg.201), published by the National Research Council.

People with this genetic disorder "therefore should greatly limit their intake of plant sterols," the article says.

As for the rest of us, many studies have shown the benefits of eating plenty of vegetables every day.

Veggies are rich in vital nutrients like vitamins A, B-complex and C, plus minerals like iron and magnesium.

In addition, plants provide fiber and several substances that seem to guard against a variety of diseases, including cancer, stroke and heart disease.

Alcohol and pain killer combo can damage liver

If you drink four or five highballs every day, don't take Tylenol for your resulting headache.

If you have an alcohol problem, taking the pain-killer acetaminophen could deliver a knock-out blow to your liver, warns a report in the *Southern Medical Journal* (83,9:1047).

Acetaminophen is a common over-the-counter pain reliever found in Tylenol, Anacin-3, Contac and more than 80 other brand-name pain relievers, cold and sinus medicines.

Doctors commonly warn people about taking too much

acetaminophen — an overdose could result in deadly liver damage.

In a new wrinkle, researchers warn that taking acetaminophen in amounts only slightly over the suggested dose could be deadly for people suffering from chronic alcoholism.

The danger lies in the combined effect of chronic alcoholism and acetaminophen. The combination actually can poison the liver. This condition is usually treatable, but it occasionally results in death.

People who drink moderate to large amounts of alcohol on a regular basis should ask their doctors about which over-the-counter pain reliever is most safe and effective for them.

'Wrinkle cream' responsible for nausea, swelling

Using a commonly prescribed facial cream threw a big wrinkle into one 64-year-old woman's hopes and plans for smoother skin.

She had been suffering from dry skin and was concerned about some increased facial wrinkling, so her doctor prescribed the cream tretinoin (also known as Retin-A), a common "wrinkle-removing" cream.

The cream worked fine for about five weeks, reports a digest in the Sept. 15, 1990 *Annals of Internal Medicine* (113,6:483).

Then, after five weeks, the woman began suffering from nausea and pelvic and breast vascular congestion (swelling). Two days later, she suffered from vaginal bleeding.

Following her doctor's advice, she stopped using the tretinoin cream immediately, and all symptoms disappeared in three days.

Cases of adverse side effects caused by the popular "wrinkle-removing" drug tretinoin are not common, but they do exist.

So, if you develop any strange and unexplained symptoms after beginning tretinoin therapy, contact your physician immediately.

Common ulcer drug triggers life-threatening case of diarrhea

A 56-year-old woman almost died recently trying to avoid a stomach ulcer.

Her doctor had prescribed an anti-ulcer drug, and two days later, she found herself in the hospital in a life-threatening situation.

A common side effect of some NSAIDs is ulcer disease, and many doctors try to avoid those ulcers by prescribing anti-ulcer medications, such as misoprostol.

However, for this 56-year-old woman, that was almost a deadly action, reports *Annals of Internal Medicine* (113,6:474).

The woman began taking misoprostol to treat the bleeding ulcers that had been caused by her NSAID therapy.

Two days after she started taking misoprostol, she developed a life-threatening case of diarrhea. She was admitted to the hospital for treatment.

The misoprostol treatment was stopped immediately, and the adverse symptoms disappeared over the next five or six days.

Apparently, the woman had a mild case of a kind of inflammatory bowel disease that had gone unnoticed for several years, and she forgot to tell her doctor about it. So, the doctor prescribed misoprostol, which aggravated the bowel disease and caused the dangerous diarrhea.

Researchers suggest that people with any form of bowel disorder should avoid misoprostol treatment.

You should also make sure your doctor knows about all illnesses or health conditions you have before he prescribes your medications. A complete health history will help him prescribe the safest and most effective medications for your needs.

Acidic foods and drinks reduce the effectiveness of nicotine gum

If you're chewing nicotine gum to help you kick the tobacco habit, think twice before you order that soft drink or put ketchup and mustard on your burger!

Foods and drinks with high acid content can actually prevent you from absorbing the nicotine from the gum, warns *The Journal of the American Medical Association* (264,12:1560).

Normally, your body easily absorbs nicotine by way of the saliva released in your mouth as you chew the gum. But when you eat acidic foods and drinks, the acidity of your saliva changes. Then you can't absorb the nicotine released from the gum.

The next problem is that the nicotine that is not absorbed in the mouth is swallowed and ends up in the stomach where it can cause some unpleasant side effects.

If you have an acidic drink or food, you can still use nicotine gum... just wait about 20 minutes. The saliva in your mouth will return to normal then, and you can get the full benefit of the nicotine gum.

The acidity of foods and drinks is measured on a pH scale of 1 to 14. The value of 7.0 is neutral. Water has a pH of about 7.0 and is neutral. All values below 7.0 are acidic — the lower the number, the more acidic it is. See the chart of food and drink pH values given below for further information about which foods and drinks to avoid while chewing nicotine gum.

Foods and drinks to avoid while using nicotine gum

Substance	pH value
Chocolate milk	6.76
Whole milk	6.72
Skim milk	6.58
Chicken soup	6.54
2% lowfat milk	6.53
Distilled water	6.02 - 7.28
Coffee	4.86 - 5.45
Tomato juice	4.37
Beer	4.00 - 4.60
Soy sauce	3.92
Apple juice	3.88
Orange juice	3.81 - 3.89
Ketchup	3.66
Pineapple juice	3.64
Mustard	3.34 - 4.87
Diet cola	3.32 - 3.36
Lemon-lime soda	3.22 - 3.28
Grape juice	3.17
Cola	2.30 - 2.76

Glaucoma drug causes taste disturbances

Has your food been tasting funny lately?

Noticed that your favorite meal no longer appeals to you?

Finding that you don't enjoy your morning coffee like you used to?

If so, you might be experiencing a taste disturbance.

If you're taking the drug acetazolamide to help manage your glaucoma and you've noticed a change in your taste, you are probably suffering from an adverse drug side effect.

Apparently, the drug acetazolamide can cause a taste disturbance that can occur as quickly as six hours after taking the first dose and last for as long as 24 hours after the last dose, reports the Nov. 11, 1990 *The Lancet* (336,8724:1190).

This little-known side effect could be serious in an indirect way.

Elderly people who are suffering from taste disturbances may begin neglecting their meals because the food doesn't taste right. This could lead to nutritional problems and vitamin deficiencies.

If you are experiencing changes in your sense of taste, do not stop taking the drug. Instead, speak to your doctor.

He may be able to prescribe another drug that will help manage your glaucoma and not interfere with your sense of taste and your eating habits.

Caution: the medications your doctor prescribed might do more harm than good

Are the medications you're taking for your health helping or hurting you?

Or, are they doing a little of both?

Medications can literally be life-savers in their ability to improve an elderly person's health. However, some medications can also seriously compromise or endanger someone's health through their bad side effects.

Bad side effects are especially common among elderly people. Due to the bodily changes that accompany aging, a healthy dose of many medications for a younger person may be too strong for an older person. For example, a 10-milligram dose of Valium for a 35-year-old man might just relax his muscles. That same dose of Valium in a 75-year-old woman would relax her muscles so much that she could lose all muscle coordination and be unable to get around, warns the November 1990 *FDA Consumer* (24,9:24).

Or, some kinds of medications that cause few or no side effects in younger people often cause a wide variety of side effects in the older population.

For instance, a simple anti-inflammatory drug could help ease the pain of aching joints without any adverse side effects in a young athlete. That same anti-inflammatory drug in an older person could help relieve the pain and stiffness of arthritis. However, it could also cause gastrointestinal irritation, ruin the appetite, and interfere with proper digestion.

In fact, two of the most common adverse side effects of many oral medications (medications taken by mouth) are digestion problems and nutritional disturbances.

Some drugs prevent vitamins and minerals from being absorbed into the body properly.

Other drugs interfere with food consumption or enjoyment by causing dry mouth or decreasing the sense of taste, reports *Geriatric Nursing* (11,6:301).

Diarrhea and constipation, as well as depression and dementia (mental confusion), are other common side effects of many medications.

A very common problem that many elderly people face is that of drug interactions.

Most elderly people take more than one kind of medication. Occasionally, these different drugs react to each other and cause negative side effects when they meet in the bloodstream or digestive system.

Another cause of negative drug side effects is improper use

of the medications. Often, many people do not fully understand the proper way to use the medication. Using some drugs at the wrong time or with the wrong kinds of food or drink can produce side effects that could be easily avoided.

If you think you are experiencing some negative side effects from one or more of your medications, talk to your doctor immediately. If you are taking prescription drugs, do not stop taking the drugs without first consulting with your physician.

The negative effects of stopping drug therapy can be much more dangerous, or even life-threatening, than any of the negative side effects you're experiencing.

So, be sure to speak with your doctor before changing your medication routine.

Here's a list of questions that may be helpful to ask the doctor:

- What is the drug I'm taking?
- What is the drug supposed to do?
- What are the possible side effects?
- Is the drug habit-forming?
- Should I take the drug with food or avoid food when I take it?
- At what times of the day should I take the drug?
- Should I avoid any activities while taking the drug, such as driving or exercising?

If you are experiencing negative side effects from one or more over-the-counter drugs, the wisest course of action is to talk with your local pharmacist.

He can suggest some other over-the-counter drugs that will perform the same service without the negative side effects.

Or, he may suggest a non-drug form of therapy for dealing with your situation.

To insure the safest and most effective use of your medications, see the following table of some "*Do*'s" and "*Don't*'s" of drug therapy.

To ensure the safest and most effective use of your medicines: Do's and Don't's

---

Do's

✔ Call your doctor immediately if you notice any new symptoms or side effects, such as confusion, sleeplessness, incontinence or impotence.

✔ Store your medicines properly. This usually means storing them in a cool, dry place. Some medicine should be stored in the refrigerator. The bathroom is usually not the best place to store drugs. Bathrooms are warm, damp places, and some drugs may lose their potency if exposed to moisture.

✔ Always read the labels and other information and instructions provided with the prescription.

✔ Always throw away old or expired medicines. Make sure you flush them down the toilet instead of throwing them into the trash can.

✔ Be sure to take the exact amount prescribed.

Don't's

✘ Do not take medicine in the dark. Always turn on the light and make sure you are taking the right medicine.

✘ Never stop taking a drug suddenly without checking with your doctor — even if you feel better.

✘ Do not take drugs prescribed for someone else or give your drug to anyone else.

✘ Don't transfer a drug from its original bottle to another.

✘ Never drink alcoholic beverages while you're taking your medication unless your doctor says it's okay. Mixing alcohol with medicine can be dangerous. Of the 100 medicines commonly prescribed, over half contain at least one substance that reacts badly with alcohol.

Drugs that interfere with nutrition

Aspirin: Interferes with levels of folic acid and ascorbic acid in the blood, and causes a deficiency of iron.

Laxatives: Interferes with the absorption of calcium in the body.

Penicillin: Reduces the amount of potassium in the body by increasing the amount of potassium released in the urine.

Mineral oil:
Interferes with the absorption of vitamins such as vitamins A, D and E.

Antacids that contain aluminum:
Reduce absorption of fluoride and phosphorus

in the body, and reduce the amount of calcium by increasing the amount of calcium lost in the urine.

Antacids with aluminum or magnesium:

Lowers the absorption of phosphorus in the body and increases the amount of phosphorus lost in the urine.

Antacids with sodium-bicarbonate:

Results in bloating due to water retention and sodium retention.

Tetracyclines:

Inhibits the absorption of vitamins such as iron, calcium, magnesium and zinc.

Corticosteroids:

Inhibits absorption of phosphorus and calcium and raises the body's need for other vitamins, such as vitamin D, folic acid and ascorbic acid.

Exercise and Fitness

Regular exercise helps fight heart-stopping blood clots

Losing weight and building stronger bones and muscles are just some of the benefits of regular exercise. Scientists have found another.

Regular exercise also helps your body fight blood clots, which can clog arteries and cause heart attack and strokes.

Dr. John Stratton presented the results of this new study at a recent meeting of the American Heart Association in New Orleans.

Regular exercise increases the body's production of tissue plasminogen activator, commonly called TPA, a protein that helps dissolve blood clots, Dr. Stratton says.

In fact, TPA is so effective in treating heart attack that scientists have found a way to produce it in the laboratory.

The drug is used to treat heart-attack victims in emergency rooms throughout the U.S. It works by dissolving clots that block arteries feeding the heart.

Dr. Stratton and his colleagues studied 20 people aged 25 to

74 before and after they had completed a six-month aerobic exercise program.

At the end of the study, "TPA levels increased by an average of 29 percent," according to a report from the American Heart Association.

Aerobic exercise includes jogging, walking and swimming — activities that cause you to "breathe hard" during a workout.

Other benefits of regular exercise include lower blood pressure and higher levels of high-density lipoprotein ("good") cholesterol, Dr. Stratton adds.

Fend off infections with moderate exercise

Walking may help your body fight off flu and other serious infectious diseases, according to new studies from Australia.

Moderate exercises like walking seem to boost the body's natural defenses against infections, reports *Medical Tribune* (31,9:9).

The boost to the immune system especially benefits the sensitive mucous membranes in the mouth, throat and breathing passages, the report says. Those are areas vulnerable to colds and influenza attacks.

Moderate exercise may trigger production of more "killer cells" in the bloodstream, the equivalent of sending more fresh "soldiers" into battle against invading disease germs, suggests Laurel Mackinnon, a professor of exercise physiology and wellness at the University of Queensland in Australia.

But the key is moderation, the report says.

Too much heavy exercise seems to have the opposite effect, cutting back numbers of immune system "soldiers," immunoglobulin A (IgA), for up to two days, says Professor Mackinnon.

That may be why very fit athletes seem to come down with

an unusually large number of upper respiratory infections following intense training, the report suggests.

Before you start or change your exercise program, be sure to check with your doctor about what exercises will be appropriate for you.

Walk away from cardiovascular disease

A comfortable pair of walking shoes just might add years to your life.

According to *Medical World News* (31,5:20), lack of physical fitness is as much a risk factor in cardiovascular disease as hypertension, high cholesterol, and cigarette smoking.

But, your physical fitness is easier for you to control and manage than high cholesterol or hypertension.

Even simple changes in your daily routine can produce a healthier heart.

A person "does not need an athletic level of fitness to get a lot of benefit in terms of preventing early death," stated Dr. Steven Blair, director of epidemiology at the Institute for Aerobics Research in Dallas, at a seminar sponsored by the American Heart Association.

Dr. Blair believes the medical profession needs to recognize that poor physical fitness is a leading cause of early death. To prove his theory, he conducted a study of 10,224 men and 3,120 women and the effects of their exercise habits.

The men and women were given treadmill tests to determine their beginning level of fitness, then divided into three categories — low, moderate or high fitness groups. The three groups were studied for about eight years. Over the eight year period, there were 240 deaths among the men and 43 deaths among the women.

Without exception, the men and women in the low fitness

categories experienced a higher death rate.

The findings even showed that exercise provided extra protection for smokers and those with higher levels of cholesterol.

Dr. Blair concludes that most men and women could reduce their risk of heart disease with the addition of very modest exercise.

He recommends walking as the exercise that is easiest to mold into your life-style.

A brisk walk for 30 to 45 minutes, six to seven times a week, is enough to maintain the fitness level needed for a healthier heart, the report says.

Personalize your walking time

As with any exercise, walking must be done regularly to get the greatest effects. Here are a few suggestions for developing a life-long habit.

1. First and foremost: Check with a doctor before establishing your walking routine!

2. If you enjoy walking with others, choose a partner who shares your interest and will help you resist the temptation to occasionally "cut your walk short."

3. If quiet moments are hard to find at your house, use your walk as special time apart from the crowd.

4. Choose a route that offers either the comfort of

familiarity, or the challenge of a different view, depending on your motivation.

5. Use a miniature tape-player to listen to music, learn a new language, or "read-a-book" from the many available selections on cassettes.

6. Make a personal commitment to "stick-to-it." It just might mean a longer life.

Choosing just the right "equipment"

Like every sport, walking requires the right equipment. But since there are no balls, bats, rackets or clubs, we often overlook the one thing that is needed — proper shoes.

Here are a few suggestions from orthopedists, podiatrists and serious walkers on how to buy shoes that will help you put your best foot forward.

1. Because it is recommended that you wear two pairs of socks (thin socks as a liner against the skin, and then a pair of thicker outer socks) to reduce friction and unwanted blisters, you should be wearing your socks when you test the new shoes for the proper fit.

2. Never shop at a store that won't let you "get the feel" of your new shoes. Take your time. Walk around the store. Make sure you have the support and flexibility you'll need to keep you walking in comfort.

3. Resist the urge to try on only one shoe. Since our

right and left feet rarely match (they're usually slightly different sizes), it's best to put on both shoes. Remember, you need enough room to wiggle your toes — all ten of them!

4. Don't shop for your shoes in the morning, since swelling feet can cause you to wear a half size larger by evening.

Finding your target heart rate and taking your pulse

To maximize your aerobic benefits from walking, it is best to find your target heart range and maintain it for at least 20 minutes.

1. Start with the number 220:   220
2. Subtract your age (50, for example):   -50
3. The answer is your maximum heart rate: 170

4. Multiply your max. heart rate by 0.6:   170
   (This is your low range; 60 percent)   x 0.6
                                                      102

5. Multiply your max. heart rate by 0.8:   170
   (This is your high range; 80 percent)   x 0.8
                                                      136

If you are a beginner, always work at the lower end of your range. Only those already physically fit should attempt to achieve the 80 percent range.

Checking your pulse is easy if you have a watch with a second hand. Place your index and middle finger along the side of your neck, just below the jaw. Count the number of beats you feel for 15 seconds, then multiply by four to arrive at your heart rate.

If you have already determined what your target heart rate should be, you can then compare your walking heart rate with the rate you hope to achieve. In this way you can keep your heart rate within safe limits without sacrificing your aerobic benefits.

Exercise is a clot buster

Ever wonder why exercise is good for your heart?

Here's one clue: Regular exercise increases the body's level of "clot dissolver," Seattle researchers reported at the annual American Heart Association meeting in New Orleans.

In their study, walking, jogging or cycling for 45 minutes "four or five times a week" increased the level of tissue plasminogen activator — the body's natural clot buster — by 39 percent in men aged 60 to 82.

Flat feet support good news

The U.S. Army and the Nike Company recently joined forces to test the time-honored belief that flat feet promote foot and leg injuries.

Surprisingly, they found that new recruits with high arches were more than twice as likely to injure their feet as trainees with flat feet.

The study suggests that the higher the arch, the higher the risk of injury, and that flat feet may prevent foot and leg injuries.

Exercise raises risk of sudden death from irregular heartbeats?

Exercisers, you may face increased danger of sudden death from irregular heartbeats.

Exercise causes irregular heartbeats? you ask. Well, not exactly.

It's not the physical activity itself that's the problem. It's the air you breathe while exercising.

You may be breathing in a variety of pollutants, including carbon monoxide and ozone.

And that could trigger skipped heartbeats or irregular heart rhythms, says a report in the September 1990 *Annals of Internal Medicine* (113,5:343). This increase in cardiac arrhythmias is dangerous because it increases a person's risk of sudden cardiac death.

These irregular heartbeats kill an estimated 350,000 people each year in the United States and represent the leading cause of sudden deaths from heart attack, says a digest in *Science News* (138,10:149).

The main sources of carbon monoxide in the environment are automobile exhaust and cigarette smoke, says an article in *The Physician and Sportsmedicine* (18,9:153).

And cigarette smoke is dangerous even if you don't smoke. Apparently, the side-stream or secondary smoke from a cigarette contains more carbon monoxide than the directly inhaled smoke.

When carbon monoxide and ozone enter the blood, they decrease the body's ability to transport oxygen effectively.

So, the heart has to work harder and beat faster to overcome the disability. This process is magnified during exercise, when the heart has to work harder anyway.

It's complicated because you absorb a lot more pollutants as you gulp in lungfuls of air during vigorous exercise.

However, the solution is not to stop exercising. In fact, deep breathing of clean air during vigorous exercising can help clear the bloodstream of carbon monoxide.

To help avoid the dangers of air pollutants, observe the safety precautions listed in "Reduce the dangers of exercise."

Reduce the dangers of exercise

■ Avoid exercising during peak traffic hours.

■ Avoid exercising in bright sunlight. Ozone levels increase on sunny days.

■ Exercise in open areas where the wind can disperse pollutants.

■ Avoid resting under trees for long periods of time. Pollutants can get trapped under trees, making shady air "dirtier."

■ Consider exercising indoors or in the country where pollutant levels are lower.

■ Avoid smoking immediately before or after exercising. If you smoke after exercising, wait until you are breathing normally.

Start jogging to boost levels of HDL cholesterol

If you have been trying to lose weight to try and control your cholesterol levels, you should consider taking up jogging. Men who have lost weight and started jogging show a marked boost in their HDL cholesterol levels, according to the Sept. 22, 1990 *Science News* (138,12:177).

HDL cholesterol is known as the "good" cholesterol, and high HDL levels help prevent coronary heart disease.

Apparently, joggers who used to be overweight enjoyed

higher HDL levels than joggers who had started out lean.

This does not mean that lean men should gain weight, then lose it, then start jogging just to get higher levels of HDL. It's simply an additional bonus for overweight men who become joggers.

Help reduce dizziness with easy exercises

You know the feeling . . . you've felt it many times before.

The room starts spinning, your head starts reeling, and you have to stop what you're doing and sit down until it passes.

Dizziness.

It's an irritating and ongoing problem that usually is caused by damage to one or both of your ears. The doctors tell you to get used to it because there's nothing you can do about it. They say the only thing you can do is avoid the motions or activities that bring on the dizziness.

That's all changed now, reports the *Medical Tribune* (31,20:2).

Doctors recently have discovered that simple home exercises can help most people control or even eliminate their dizziness.

The best time to start exercises for dizziness is right after your ears are injured.

Your ear doctor can test you for dizziness and choose special exercises for you to do at home. The exercises may be as simple as tilting your head from side to side as you sit in a chair, alternating standing on one foot at a time and then the other, or passing a ball back and forth above your head.

These exercises help reduce dizziness and increase physical strength.

Although the exercises are not considered a cure, they may be the very best way for you to manage your dizziness and get back into a normal routine.

Chronic Fatigue Syndrome: exercise to get rid of fatigue?

It's hard to pinpoint, and even harder to treat. But fatigue is almost as rampant as the "common cold."

Millions of people pay for yearly visits to their doctors, complaining of vague forms of fatigue — everything from loss of concentration to low energy levels that persist in spite of adequate rest.

Chronic Fatigue Syndrome (CFS) has been linked most often to the mononucleosis and Epstein-Barr viruses.

But recent studies seem to suggest that CFS has been around for many years, often changing names, but presenting its sufferers with the same problems.

The routine advice given to CFS patients has been to rest. But now a new approach is being tried, and it shows great promise, reports the August 1990 *Drug Therapy* (20,8:29).

Carefully planned, regular exercise — instead of an inactive life-style — is now being recommended.

The idea is to break the vicious cycle of fatigue and its inevitable results of poor fitness and poor cardiovascular health.

CFS sufferers are warned not to expect immediate results, but to gradually increase their activity until a level of fitness is achieved that cancels out most of the symptoms of fatigue.

As with most problems, a healthy diet plays an important role in recovery.

The American Heart Association recommends a low-fat diet as a wise choice. This provides your heart with the proper fuel to do its job, while supplying much-needed energy to tired muscles.

As frustrating as it might be, people experiencing CFS can bring about healthy results if they maintain a positive attitude and follow their doctor's suggestions completely.

Eyesight

Caffeine may complicate eye problems

Coffee drinkers, beware! That third cup of caffeinated coffee may be affecting your vision.

Researchers at the University of Texas and Emory University found that the caffeine in coffee can increase pressure in your eyes, which can aggravate problems related to glaucoma.

The first two cups of coffee don't seem to bother the eyes. It's the third, fourth and fifth cups that cause problems.

So people with glaucoma-related eye problems should limit their coffee intake to two cups or less each day, the report suggests.

Set a date to save your sight

Have you looked at a calendar lately?

If you're over fifty, there's more reason to look at your calendar than just to remember an important date!

Looking at the grid pattern on your calendar can reveal

important changes in your vision that may actually help you save your sight.

After you reach 50, an important part of your eye called the macula may begin to break down a little bit. The macula is located at the back of your eye in the center of the retina, and it is the area of your eye that is most sensitive to light.

If the macula deteriorates, the middle of your field of vision becomes blurred or dark. This condition is called age-related macular degeneration (AMD). According to *Health After 50* (2,2:2), it affects about 25 percent of people over age 65 and 33 percent of those over 80 years.

If you have AMD, you may notice blurring or haziness in the center of your vision. Straight lines may look wavy, and you may not see colors as well as you used to. Fortunately, most people do not have serious vision loss from AMD.

However, people with AMD have about a 10 percent chance of developing a more serious condition called "wet" AMD. In wet AMD, tiny blood vessels at the back of the eye begin to leak, causing scarring and loss of central vision.

Health After 50 reports that wet AMD may develop suddenly at any time and cause rapid and severe vision loss within days or weeks.

This is where your calendar comes in. By monitoring your vision regularly, you can detect changes in it early enough to see your ophthalmologist right away and stop the damage caused by wet AMD.

Your doctor can give you an Amsler grid that looks much like a calendar to use when checking your vision.

Cover one eye and look at the Amsler grid or a calendar to see if the area on which you are focusing is clear or distorted. Then cover the other eye and check it.

If the center of the grid pattern looks broken, distorted or wavy to either eye, visit your doctor right away. An ophthalmologist can use laser treatment to stop these vessels from leaking and slow down the progress of wet AMD.

People suffering from AMD often are declared "legally blind" (less than 20/200 vision), says *The Merck Manual* (15th edition). However, these people usually have good peripheral vision and useful color vision, and they should be reassured that they won't lose all their vision.

There's no cure for AMD yet. But you can do two things to protect yourself from this cause of blindness.

See your eye doctor every year, and check your eyes with a calendar or an Amsler grid regularly. It could save you from serious vision loss.

(For information on low-vision aid devices, write to American Foundation for the Blind Consumer Products Division, 15 West 16th Street, New York, NY 10011.)

Contaminated mascara blinds Georgia woman

A 47-year-old Georgia woman was blinded when she accidentally scratched her cornea as she was applying mascara, her doctors report in *The Journal of the American Medical Association* (263,12:1616).

She complained of "pain, light sensitivity, redness and swelling of the eye," according to their report. She was given an eye ointment, and the eye was patched.

Three days later, the woman's conditioned worsened. She developed an infection in her eye and her vision was severely impaired. Doctors admitted her to the hospital.

After treatment, the infection cleared up, but the woman failed to regain her sight.

The woman lost her sight because her mascara was contaminated with the bacteria, *Pseudomonas aeruginosa*. The report points out that "new mascara is rarely contaminated with bacteria but can become contaminated . . . after use."

The lesson: Don't use a tube of mascara for more than a few months, and always apply make-up carefully. If you suffer *any* type of eye injury, see your doctor right away.

Vitamins help slash risk of cataracts

People who take regular daily doses of either vitamin C or vitamin E may slash by more than half their risk of developing blinding cataracts, according to a report in *Science News* (135,20:308).

Scientists don't know for sure why the vitamins prevent cloudy formations in aging eyes. Some researchers believe that vitamins C and E, both of which are antioxidants, neutralize damaging lens proteins before they can clump together.

But too much of a good thing can be harmful.

Check with your doctor before taking either of these nutrients.

Cataracts' triggers include sunlight, diabetes and steroids.

Sun lovers more prone to cataracts

The more time you spend in the sun, the greater your risk of developing cataracts, researchers report in *Good Health Bulletin* (II,3:3).

Golfers, sailors and gardeners, for example, are exposed to more ultraviolet (UV) radiation than usual and should always wear sunglasses when outdoors — even on cloudy days.

Look for sunglasses that block 100 percent of UV radiation.

Avoid dangerous look-alikes that may cause serious eye injuries

Before you apply your eye drops, double check that bottle — you could be making a sticky mistake!

The glue containers in "do-it-yourself" artificial nail kits are often identical to bottles used for prescription eye drops.

As a result, *The Journal of the American Medical Association* (263,17:2301) reports than an increasing number of people mistakenly apply glue to their eyes instead of medicine, causing painful injuries.

You can avoid a mix-up by taking the following precautions: try putting colorful labels on glue containers, eye drops and other medicine bottles to help you tell them apart.

You may also find it helpful to store glue and nail kits separately from your medicine.

Watch the clock for best eye therapy results

High noon used to be the best showdown time for gunfighters in Western movies. High noon also seems to be the best time to put eyedrops in your eyes.

If you're using prescription eyedrops to help treat your glaucoma, watching the clock makes a big difference in how effective your treatment is.

Researchers are finding that eyedrop drug therapy may be most effective at certain times of the day and less effective at other times.

Using the glaucoma eyedrops at special times in the day may increase the effectiveness of the drug and cut down on the adverse side-effects at the same time, according to a report in the Sept. 6, 1990 issue of *Medical Tribune* (31,18:4).

Researchers used lab animals to test the effectiveness of timolol (a common glaucoma drug) at 6 a.m., noon, 6 p.m. and midnight.

They found the drug to be most effective, with the fewest bad side-effects, at noon.

Human testing is on the way. Researchers are excited about improving glaucoma treatment just by keeping an eye on the clock.

For safety's sake, don't change your eyedrop schedule without checking with your doctor first.

Health Tips

Drink more water to fight confusion

Some of the symptoms can be similar to those of dementia. That's the dreaded senility and destruction of the mind that comes with Alzheimer's disease and some kinds of strokes.

It's a serious situation, but, in some cases, it can be cured just by drinking water, according to reports in *Gerontological Nursing* (16,5:4) and *Senior Health Digest* (June 30, 1990; pg.3).

Simple dehydration — loss of too much of the body's water supply — can bring on mental confusion, disorientation, seizures and other problems.

As many as four out of 10 elderly people admitted to hospitals for dehydration die from complications brought on by fluid loss.

The treatment is fairly simple: drink lots of fluids, especially water, at least two-and-a-half pints daily, says the report.

Some seniors stay in a constant state of dehydration, simply because their mouths don't tell them that they need water. They don't feel thirsty even though their bodies may be suffering from lack of fluids.

The thirst response gets rusty with increased age, lagging by two or three days.

In other words, your body might need water on Monday, but you might not get the thirst message until Wednesday.

That's bad any time of year, but hot weather raises the danger level.

During hot weather, you need to drink more fluids to keep your body properly cooled and to make up for fluid lost in sweating.

In addition, blood flow to the skin can be 50 percent lower in people over 65, says the *Digest*. That further lowers the body's cooling ability.

To be on the safe side, suggests *New Health Tips Encyclopedia* (FC&A, 1989; pg.13), drink enough fluids to keep the urine a pale yellow in color, not dark. Dark or cloudy urine might indicate you're not getting enough water.

During hot weather, weigh yourself daily, and drink a pint of water for every pound that you lose, whether you feel thirsty or not, researchers suggest.

Check with your doctor about your fluid needs and how best to meet them.

Suffering from dry mouth?

It could be caused from using snuff or chewing tobacco.

People who use smokeless tobacco have a lot of saliva when they are using the tobacco. But they have a lower-than-normal amount of saliva in their mouths when they are not using it.

Researchers from Emory University believe that the increased dryness may lead to more plaque on the teeth, which can cause tooth decay, says a report in *News Tips From Emory University* (April-May 1989).

Aspirin therapy for migraine headaches

If you're one of the millions of Americans who suffer migraine headaches, a small daily dose of aspirin may relieve your pain, Boston researchers reported at a recent American Heart Association conference.

In an eight-year study, 22,000 male doctors aged 40 to 84 took either 325 milligrams of aspirin or a placebo without aspirin every day to test how aspirin helps fight heart disease.

During this heart disease study, scientists accidentally discovered that aspirin also helped relieve the doctors' migraine symptoms, such as nausea, light sensitivity and severe pain on one side of the head.

In a follow-up questionnaire, 840 people taking the placebo had migraines, compared with only 672 taking aspirin — a 20 percent difference.

Although the findings are encouraging, Harvard University Professor Julie E. Buring says, "I think migraine [headache] requires much more study. It's not clear what triggers [it]."

Researchers still don't know why an "ordinary" headache progresses to a more painful migraine.

Re-leaf for headache pain

Using herbal "medicines" to relieve common aches and pains is not just old folklore. Some scientists say that herbs may be just as helpful and useful in treating illnesses as modern medicine.

One such herb, called feverfew, may help cut the number and severity of migraine headaches you've been experiencing.

A digest report in *Science News* (134:106) suggests that taking daily capsules of ground feverfew leaves reduces migraine headache discomfort and also helps relieve the nausea that sometimes accompanies migraine headaches.

However, you should check with your doctor before trying any herbal supplement.

Avoid painful infections easily

Douching regularly may bring on painful infections, reports *The Journal of the American Medical Association* (263,14:1936).

Researchers studied a group of women who routinely douche once a week.

This group was nearly four times as likely to come down with pelvic inflammatory disease as women who douche less than once a month.

Many women rinse out the vaginal canal following sexual relations or as part of ordinary hygiene.

That might be medically unsafe for some, suggests the Seattle study of 1,000 women.

Why? Because douching might flush out protective bacteria and introduce harmful germs, the scientists speculate.

Curiously, women had more problems with PID using disposable bottles of commercially-prepared douching solutions.

Women had fewer infections when they used plain water or homemade water-plus-vinegar solutions, the report says.

PID is a severe infection of the reproductive tract. It sometimes causes sterility or abscesses. Infected abscesses may rupture, and require immediate surgery.

Change in life-style can create a longer life span

Middle-aged men who adopt healthy life-style changes can greatly reduce their risk of dying from a heart attack a decade later.

High blood pressure, high cholesterol, and smoking are known risk factors for heart disease, but they don't have to end your life. Beginning a program of intervention aimed at halting the consequences of heart disease may just help save your life!

The Multiple Risk Factor Intervention Trial (MRFIT) was set up to determine the effects of life-style changes in men who fit the high risk category of coronary heart disease.

According to *The Journal of the American Medical Association* (263,13:1795), researchers at the University of Minnesota in Minneapolis conducted a 10.5 year study to determine the benefits derived from an intervention program designed to overturn the negative effects of life-styles that promote heart disease.

The MRFIT program consisted of over 12,000 men, aged 35 to 57, all fitting the high risk requirements. These men were divided into two categories — those in the intervention program and those using only their private medical care (no extra intervention).

The intervention program, with a total of 6,428 men, involved diet changes to lower cholesterol levels, counseling to stop smoking, and any necessary treatment to control high blood pressure. The 6,438 remaining men received no special instructions, but used their normal sources of health care.

During the decade following the onset of the program, the value of intervention became obvious. The cardiovascular disease mortality rate was 8.3 percent lower in the group that received special instructions.

In narrowing the analysis to fatal heart attacks, the researchers found a 24 percent drop in deaths among the intervention group compared to the usual-care group.

Change can be difficult, but when the benefits include a longer and more productive life, the effort seems worthwhile.

Ask your doctor if a diet lower in saturated fats and cholesterol, medication or exercise to lower your blood pressure, and a program to stop smoking, would take you out of the "high risk" category.

Swimmer's ear can spoil summer fun

Imagine you're at the beach. The weather is perfect, and you've been swimming every day. Then one of your grandchildren complains that her ear feels itchy and sore. When you touch the ear or she moves her jaw from side to side, the pain is worse.

It's likely that she has a bacterial infection called otitis externa, or swimmer's ear, and she'll have to stay out of the water until it's cleared up.

Swimmer's ear can happen to anyone, but it happens most often to people who get moisture in their ears during water activities. When water stays in your ears, it breaks down the protective covering in the ear canal, and sets up the perfect conditions for bacteria to grow.

People get swimmer's ear for other reasons, too. Some people's ears are formed so that debris and water accumulate in the outer ear canal, encouraging bacterial growth. Also, people who have certain skin conditions tend to get swimmer's ear more often.

U.S. Pharmacist (15,5:73) advises that swimmer's ear can usually be cured in the early stages with non-prescription ear drops containing alcohol and acetic acid. If a more serious infection develops, you will need to see your doctor for treatment and antibiotic ear drops.

However, if you keep the outer ear as dry as possible, you will probably be able to avoid swimmer's ear, even if you swim frequently.

Never clean or dry your ears with cotton-tipped applicators.

They may push debris deeper into the ear or damage the lining of your outer ear canal, making it easier for bacteria to grow.

To get the water out of your ears after water sports, shake your head vigorously or tilt your head to the side and jump up and down. You can also fan your ears or blow them dry with a hair dryer set on a very low temperature.

Finally, use a trick practiced by competitive swimmers: after every swim, put three to six drops of an alcohol-acetic solution into each ear. You can buy these drops at your drugstore without a prescription.

Remember, keep your ears dry so that swimmer's ear doesn't interrupt your aquatic fun this summer.

Is man's best friend really his dog?

Pets are part of the American way of life. A wagging tail or a loving purr means unconditional love to millions of avid pet owners across the country.

Pets are given credit for longer life among persons with heart disease, greater self-sufficiency for psychiatric patients and the development of social skills among children. But according to a report in *FDA Consumer* (24,3:28-31), some pets have more to offer than devotion.

"Zoonoses" is a modern term for an age-old problem. It identifies diseases capable of being passed from animals to humans. The ancient Greeks realized the connection between rabies and dogs and the bubonic plague was transmitted to all Europe because of flea-infested rodents.

Now, thanks to improved technology, most animal-transmitted diseases are documented and studied. Once identified, most zoonoses can either be prevented or treated.

The best way to avoid problems with zoonoses is to simply

be aware of the dangers.

1. Toxicare Canis, also known as roundworm, is a parasite carried by nursing dogs and their puppies. Some estimates say that virtually every puppy has roundworm. In fact, the dog roundworm is so well established that roundworm-free puppies can only be found in litters where several generations have been raised in isolation.

Since children and puppies just naturally go together, children are prime candidates for roundworm. Coming in contact with soil contaminated with the feces of an infected dog spreads the disease. When a human becomes infected, he experiences fever, headache, cough and poor appetite.

Your veterinarian can advise you on the best steps to take for your dog or puppies to help keep roundworm from being a health problem.

2. Toxoplasmosis, a feline-related disease, is capable of living in many different animals. The one-celled animal, Toxoplasma gondii, is a parasite found in cat feces or dirt contaminated with cat feces. The cat is infected while doing what cats do best — killing and eating small rodents.

Human infection actually comes through a chain of events ending at the dinner table. When infected cats deposit their feces in pastures where cows and sheep graze, the livestock become infected. When the meat from these animals is eaten raw or undercooked, the parasite is passed on to people.

Symptoms of toxoplasmosis infection in humans can include fever, headache, swollen lymph glands, cough, sore throat, nasal congestion, loss of appetite and skin rash. Many people have immune systems strong enough to fight off the infection, but there are several categories of people that need to be especially careful of contamination.

Anyone with immune system defects or anyone receiving immunosuppressive therapy need special care to keep the disease from becoming particularly dangerous. Expectant women, especially in their first trimester, should never clean a cat's litter box or eat raw or rare meat, since toxoplasmosis can cause miscarriage, premature births, or blindness in unborn children.

3. Ringworm is not really a parasite, but a skin disease caused by a fungus. A variety of animals (including dogs, cows and horses) can carry the disease to humans. But the most likely culprit is your adorable, long-haired kitten. The ringworm fungus infects the hair of the cat and is passed on when someone pets the kitty.

In humans, the fungus usually appears on exposed parts of the body or scalp as an inflamed, scaly lesion. Your doctor can make a definite diagnosis using an ultraviolet light known as Wood's lamp. If the suspected fungus is indeed ringworm, the infected hairs will appear green under the light.

Your veterinarian can take care of your pet. Your doctor can take care of you — most doctors prescribe an iodine-based soap for infected humans.

4. Psittacosis, also known as parrot fever, is a bacterial disease affecting the bird families. Pigeons, ducks, turkeys, chickens and parrots are the best known carriers of parrot fever, although there are 130 species of domestic and wild birds that carry the bacteria.

The disease is usually transmitted to humans through contact with the feces or dust from the feathers of parrots or parakeets.

People with parrot fever usually suffer from respiratory problems, such as cough and chest pain. They can also have fever, chills, vomiting and muscular pain.

An infected bird may have poor eating habits or droopy feathers, but sometimes they exhibit no symptoms at all. The best precaution is to wear a surgical or dust mask and rubber gloves while cleaning your bird's cage. If you have reason to suspect you have the disease, a blood test can determine for sure if you have psittacosis. Fortunately, antibiotics are effective in treating both humans and birds.

5. Lyme disease, named after the town of Old Lyme, Conn., was identified in the mid-1970's. However, it hasn't been confined to that area.

Deer ticks are the carriers of Lyme disease. These tiny ticks, no larger than a pin-head, attach themselves to white-tailed deer, field mice and other wild animals whose bodies contain the bacteria known as Borrelia burgdorferi. After becoming infected with the host's blood, the tick moves on to other animals or humans and infects them.

Deer ticks can attach themselves directly to you, or they can enter your home on your dog. Checking your dog for ticks after a day in heavy growth is always advisable. Since deer ticks are so small, they can be "rolled-away" with roller-type lint removers if they aren't attached.

Doctors use a blood test to help diagnose Lyme disease.

Symptoms of Lyme disease are vague and numerous, but generally the first sign is a bull's eye rash. Some people experience flu-like symptoms in the joints, chronic fatigue, dizziness, shortness of breath and a rash. Antibiotics in the early stages are absolutely necessary to prevent more serious problems (such as arthritis and cardiac/nervous disorders) that have been associated with untreated Lyme disease.

6. Rocky Mountain Spotted Fever is primarily carried by the American dog tick. The infected tick that carries the disease can be found in the woods or on your friendly pooch.

Since the tick carrying Rocky Mountain Spotted Fever is much larger than the deer tick, it is much easier to locate — on your dog and on you. Wearing long sleeves, pants and a hat when walking in heavily wooded areas will give you a measure of protection against any tick latching on. Always check yourself and your dog for any "hitch-hikers" immediately after your outing.

Symptoms of Rocky Mountain Spotted Fever are similar to those from other illnesses and include headache, fever and skin rash. Early diagnosis and antibiotic treatment is necessary to prevent serious consequences.

7. Rabies is a deadly virus transmitted by an infected animal. Left unattended, rabies is deadly. If you are bitten by an animal (wild or tame) that is possibly rabid, cleanse the wound immediately with a strong stream of water, soap or detergent, and a solution of alcohol or iodine. Then, and most important, see a doctor immediately. A series of rabies shots could save your life.

8. Cat Scratch Fever is an infection from a cat scratch or bite. What causes a particular scratch or bite to become infected isn't really understood. The sore is slow to heal, and after several months, your lymph nodes may swell and become tender and painful. This disease is uncomfortable, but seldom serious. If the problem is still uncorrected after three weeks, you should see a physician to determine if medication is needed.

Another problem among pet owners is the concern over common infections being passed from human to pet to human. Dr. Isadore Rosenfeld, clinical professor of medicine in the cardiology division of New York Hospital-Cornell Medical Center, sites an example where a family with children might be plagued constantly with sore throats. When throat cultures are done, the results show strep throat, which is treated immediately with medication. The children are cured, only to find that within a few weeks everyone is sick again. Finally, someone thinks to check the throat of the family dog and finds the dog has been the carrier of the bacteria all along.

Salmonella, a bacteria that causes mild to severe inflammation of the stomach and intestines, diarrhea and vomiting, can be passed from animals to humans. It is a serious matter for very young children, the elderly or anyone with an impaired immune system.

Dogs and birds can carry Salmonella, but turtles pose a special risk. In fact, in 1975, the FDA found "pet-sized" turtles to be such a health problem that they banned the sale of any turtle with a shell length less than four inches.

Turtles should be excluded when thinking of pets, since those in the wild are just as likely to have Salmonella as the pet store varieties.

Proper Choice of Pets

Although risks are involved, most pet owners agree that the good times outweigh the bad. Consider following a few tips when selecting a pet:

* Always choose a healthy pet — avoid dull coats, drooping feathers, or lifeless, always-sleepy animals. If in doubt about the behavior of certain species, check with your vet.

* Look at the cages or pens where your would-be pet is living prior to living with you. How clean are the surroundings? If you are buying from a pet store, are you satisfied with the appearance of the other animals they sell? Chances are, if the rabbits aren't in good shape, the parrots probably won't be either.

* Arrange for a vet to check over your new family member as soon as possible. Certain animals need vaccines, and others need care that only a veterinarian could advise.

* Once the pet becomes your responsibility, you would be wise to follow a schedule of inoculations and routine check-ups for parasites.

* Keep all cages and pens clean and free from bacteria by removing droppings and solid waste as soon as possible. Don't use pet waste as fertilizer — you could be spreading disease.

* Check for ticks and mites often, especially in the summer months.

* Never feed raw meat to your pets.

* Teach children to never pet or handle sick or strange animals. Also consider a good hand-washing routine procedure after handling any animal.

* Keep your child's sandbox covered to discourage neighborhood cats from using it as a litter box.

Enjoying your pet doesn't have to be a hazard to your health. Use common sense and professional advice to help your pet be a pleasant and safe part of your family.

Life-threatening blood infection from deer ticks

Another dangerous disease from the deer tick — This time it's a life-threatening blood infection called babesiosis.

A 63-year-old Wisconsin woman was sick for a month with fever, chills, headaches, extreme tiredness and jaundice, a yellowing of the skin caused by a liver problem. Earlier, she had been treated for Lyme disease

Doctors believe she was bitten by a tick that had earlier bitten an animal infected with babesiosis.

The same tick bite that caused the Lyme disease also might have carried the Babesia germ as well, says Dr. Vincent Iacopino in *Archives of Internal Medicine* (150,7:1527).

Because of a long incubation period, it took many months for the babesiosis to make her sick.

The woman required breathing help from a ventilator until intense treatment with an antibiotic, quinine and a nearly complete exchange of blood by transfusions.

Babesiosis has been rare in the U.S.A., but this report says more cases may show up in the northern Midwest.

Deer ticks are about the size of a pencil point, making them hard to see.

Prevent tick bites by wearing clothing that covers completely.

Apply insect repellent before going outside, and take a shower immediately after returning from woods or areas where wild animals might have been.

Pollution slows body's defenses

Researchers at the University of Southern California caution that nitrogen dioxide, a common pollutant from auto exhaust, appears to damage lung cells and tissues. The damage makes the lungs more susceptible to cancer growth, says a report in *Science News* (137,14:221).

Nitrogen dioxide also damages the body's natural "killer"

cells that help the immune system fight off other sicknesses.

Licorice lovers alert

Those who like a bit of licorice candy every day may be left with a bad taste in their mouths.

Adults who eat licorice every day run a higher than normal risk of developing high blood pressure and heart disease.

According to a report in *The New England Journal of Medicine* (322,12:849), licorice causes the body to store excess salt, which in turn raises blood pressure and puts a strain on the heart.

Researchers recommend that licorice lovers cut way back on their treat and eat it only on special occasions.

Fast-food flare-up

The skin rashes and acne problems you have today may have been caused by the hamburger and French fries you ate last night.

Many fast-food restaurants serve meals in which the iodine content of each meal is 30 times the Recommended Dietary Allowance for iodine, says *The New England Journal of Medicine* (322,8:558).

The excess iodine can interfere with thyroid functions, causing rashes and acne. To avoid these flare-ups, eat fast-food only occasionally, not every day, the researchers suggest.

Natural appetite suppressant

If you want to lose weight, but have difficulty curbing your appetite, a glass of fruit juice may be just what you need.

According to a recent report in *The American Journal of Clinical Nutrition* (51,3:428), fructose, the natural sugar in fruit, is three to four times more effective in suppressing the appetite as glucose.

Studies showed that people who drank a glucose-sweetened drink about 40 minutes before each meal ate 10 to 15 percent fewer calories than those who just drank water before the meal.

However, those who drank fructose-sweetened juices ate 20 to 40 percent fewer calories at the next meal. So, try a glass of fructose-sweetened fruit juice about 45 minutes before lunch to curb your appetite and help you lose weight.

Tired of puffy eyes?

If you've been getting plenty of sleep, and your eyes still have dark rings around them or look puffy, it could be because of the way you sleep.

Sleeping on your stomach can cause normal body fluids to pool in your eye tissues. Your unseen enemy is gravity.

The extra fluid is not dangerous; it just gives you the puffy-eyed look.

To avoid this problem, try sleeping on your back with an extra pillow under your head to keep your face and eyes free from fluid build-up.

Dieters' blues

If you're tempted to eat everything in sight each time you open the refrigerator, try a blue bulb. The color blue often helps curb an overactive appetite, says a digest in *Vitality* (4,3:N6).

Installing a blue light bulb in your refrigerator may help curb your appetite and prevent you from eating yourself out of house and home.

I beg your pardon

If you're finding yourself having to ask people to repeat themselves more and more often because of a slight hearing loss, you may need to check your diet.

Too much fat in the diet can clog tiny arteries in your ears, say researchers at Mercy Hospital in Rockville Centre, New York. The clogged arteries in your ears may result in a slight loss of hearing.

Fish and rice

Recent research shows that rice bran plus fish oil appears to reduce fat in the blood better than wheat bran plus fish oil.

According to a report in *The Journal of Nutrition* (120,4:325), rice bran plus fish oil does a better job of cutting blood cholesterol.

So, if you're watching your diet to lower your cholesterol, try some tuna and rice.

Women, count your teeth

Swedish researchers are urging dentists to be on the look-out for warning signs of osteoporosis. Recent studies reported in the *British Medical Journal* (300,6730:1024) have shown that the fewer teeth women have, the greater their chances of developing brittle-bone disease.

Women should ask their dentists to be alert for two warning signs — loss of teeth and gum disease (problems with the tissues around the teeth).

If these conditions are present, women should consult their doctors about osteoporosis risks.

"Take only at meal times"

How closely you follow the directions on your medicine bottles will determine how effective your medicines will be.

Food can either help or hurt the effectiveness of the medications. So, medications that should be taken with food are obviously most effective when taken with food.

When taken on an empty stomach, the medications don't work as well. And medications that should *not* be taken with food lose some of their effectiveness if taken on a full stomach, reports *The Lancet* (335,8689:597).

If you have questions about when or how to take your medicine, be sure to contact your doctor or pharmacist immediately. It could make the difference between sickness and health for you.

Milk causes cataracts?

That second bowl of ice cream after supper could be increasing your risks of cataracts, warn researchers in *Science News* (137,12:189).

The danger lies in the milk sugar galactose, which is found in most dairy products. This kind of milk sugar may hurt the lens of the eye if the sugar is not properly digested.

People who lack the ability to break down galactose run a four times greater risk of developing cataracts than those who digest it normally.

Even people who consume small amounts of dairy products risk cataract development if they cannot metabolize milk sugars. Ask your doctor about your chances of developing cataracts from dairy products.

Vitamins and nerve damage

If you've been experiencing weakness, loss of sensory abilities, confusion and a tendency to stumble and fall, you may be short on vitamin B12.

Researchers in *U.S. Pharmacist* (15,3:78) report that these symptoms may be caused by a vitamin B12 deficiency and could result in damage to the nervous system.

However, nervous system damage can easily be avoided by eating more foods rich in vitamin B12 or with vitamin supplements to complement the diet.

Check with your doctor before you begin eating larger amounts of vitamin B12. Too much can be as dangerous as too little!

This 'hot' cream gives pain relief

For people who haven't been able to find relief from the pain and discomfort of diabetic neuropathy and pain after surgery, scientists have a "new" remedy.

The "new" is actually a reproduction of the old, only a little stronger and more effective. The new remedy is a stronger formula of non-prescription capsaicin cream.

Capsaicin is made from one of the natural ingredients that makes peppers hot.

According to an August news digest in *Geriatrics* (45,8:19), most people who use the new, stronger cream report improvements in sleeping, walking, working and recreation.

The only drawback — capsaicin may cause stinging and redness of the skin for the first few days of use. However, those minor problems disappear within three or four days.

An extra benefit is that capsaicin gets into the skin but not into your system, so it is safe to use even if you are taking several other medications, says the report.

Cool relief for headache pain

If you have frequent headaches, or even migraines, a recent article in *Modern Medicine* (58,4:84) suggests that a cold pack on your head could be your key to relief.

The results of a study done at a headache clinic indicate that using an ice pack in addition to the usual medicine helped most people feel better.

Check with your doctor: 20 or 30 minutes of cold pack treatment could be the remedy you've been looking for.

Are there hidden dangers in your mouth?

What's in your mouth might cause you to start feeling down in the mouth.

Those silver fillings in your teeth contain one of the most poisonous "heavy" metals known, and some dentists are beginning to worry about the long-term risks, cautions an article in the Sept. 18, 1990 issue of *The Atlanta Journal* (A11).

The potential danger is this: the fillings are not 100 percent silver. Silver is relatively harmless.

The fillings are made of silver "amalgam," a mixture that is about 50 percent mercury. The chemical and physical processes that produce amalgam are supposed to keep mercury locked into the tooth and away from your tissues.

However, a small but growing number of scientists believe that mercury in tooth fillings can "leak" into the tissues in the mouth in dangerous amounts and then spread to other parts of the body.

"Fillings release small amounts of mercury into the body, particularly when the amalgam is new," cautions Dr. Miroslav Marek, a researcher at the Georgia Institute of Technology.

"It is quite clear that the highest amount of mercury is released during and immediately following the actual filling of the cavity," he warns. "There is a question about what happens during those peaks of exposure, as the body absorbs the mercury, distributes it to various organs."

In addition to the immediate danger associated with new fillings, there is also a concern about mercury being released over longer periods of time.

The filling is covered with a layer of tin — part of the amalgam material—which prevents the mercury from "leaking" into the tissues in the mouth, Dr. Marek explains.

However, this film of tin can be damaged or destroyed over

time by chewing and other abrasive actions. When the protective layer of tin is damaged, mercury can escape, he argues.

Autopsy studies in Sweden and California show that mercury levels in the brain appear to be linked to the number of silver amalgam fillings in the mouth, the report in the *Journal* states.

Researchers are also finding that when mercury does "leak" from fillings, it accumulates in the highest levels in the liver and kidneys.

Some of the side effects of mercury poisoning include insomnia, slurred speech, brain damage, deafness, blindness and muscle tremors.

The alternatives to amalgam fillings are gold, porcelain, and plastic-quartz-mix fillings.

These materials cost more and aren't as easy to work with as amalgam.

The jury is still out on whether "leaky" fillings pose a measurable danger to significant numbers of people.

In the meantime, if you have unexplained symptoms that match those of mercury poisoning, ask your doctor about tests and treatments available.

Painting your walls could poison you

Finally getting around to repainting your kitchen? Well, you might want to reconsider.

It seems that many researchers are painting a pretty dangerous picture of some interior latex paints, especially those produced before August 1990.

Some brands of interior water-based latex paint contain dangerous levels of the element mercury — one of the most poisonous substances known to man.

Using these brands for painting in your house might result in

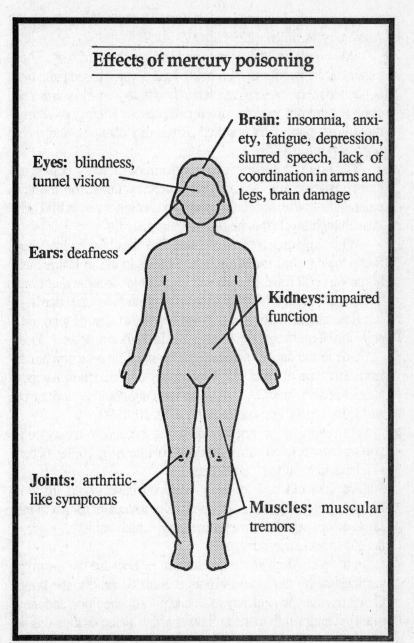

Effects of mercury poisoning

Brain: insomnia, anxiety, fatigue, depression, slurred speech, lack of coordination in arms and legs, brain damage

Eyes: blindness, tunnel vision

Ears: deafness

Kidneys: impaired function

Joints: arthritic-like symptoms

Muscles: muscular tremors

mercury poisoning, reports the Oct. 18, 1990 *New England Journal of Medicine* (323,16:1096).

One family in Michigan found this out the hard way. They repainted the interior of their house with a water-based paint that contained mercury. Ten days later, their four-year-old son developed leg cramps, a generalized rash, severe itching, sweating, rapid heart rate, fever, marked personality changes, and other serious symptoms.

The boy was suffering from a form of mercury poisoning known as acrodynia. He had inhaled mercury fumes from the new paint in his house, and the mercury had accumulated in his body in such high levels that he became seriously ill.

When researchers investigated the family's house, they found the concentration of mercury fumes in the air inside their home was 600 times the amount in the outdoor air at that time. That concentration is far greater than health safety standards.

Researchers warn that this can happen to anyone who uses any kind of mercury-containing paint in the home or workplace.

Due to the danger associated with inhaling mercury fumes from this type of paint, the Environmental Protection Agency announced on June 29, 1990, that mercury could no longer be added to interior latex paints after Aug. 20, 1990.

However, you're not safe quite yet, because mercury-containing interior latex paints produced before Aug. 20, 1990, can still be sold legally to consumers.

And the old cans of paint that you have stored in your basement or garage to touch up nicks or to repaint rooms in the same color may also contain mercury, which could pose great danger to you and your family.

Young children are in greater danger because the mercury particles in the fumes and vapors eventually settle to the floor. Children have the tendency to sit and play on the floor, and they often put their hands in their mouths, which increases their risk of mercury-poisoning.

Some scientists believe that it takes about seven years for all the mercury-containing fumes from these paints to fall to safe levels. Some studies have shown that exposure to mercury could be responsible for neurological problems such as headaches, tremors, short-term memory problems and depression.

However, there is some good news. Opening windows and doors and increasing the ventilation inside the house can help disperse the mercury fumes. Proper ventilation can reduce the fumes to a safe level in the house. But make sure you open the windows regularly for a while after painting to ensure that poisonous levels of mercury fumes don't build up inside the house again.

Another tip: when you buy new paint, make sure it was produced after Aug. 20, 1990. Avoiding mercury-containing paints altogether is your safest bet.

Aluminum and cast iron pots and pans are safe

You recently purchased a set of nonstick Teflon-coated pots and pans, and so far you have loved cooking with them! You use less oil when cooking, and cleaning is a snap.

But, you just scratched the bottom of one of the pots, and now you're concerned about the scratched Teflon contaminating your food.

Well, the Food and Drug Administration advises you not to worry.

Lately, consumers have been panicking about contaminants "leaking" into their food from their pots and pans. They have been especially worried about aluminum leaking into their food due to the distant link between aluminum and Alzheimer's disease.

However, the FDA says these fears are unfounded, reports

the October 1990 *FDA Consumer* (24, 8:12).

In response to consumers' questions, the FDA researched the following kinds of cookware: nonstick Teflon coated, anodized aluminum, regular aluminum, stainless steel, copper, cast iron, ceramic and enameled cookware.

Based on their findings, the FDA reports that most pots and pans do not "leak" — no substances from the pot or pan are absorbed by the food.

However, a few types of pots and pans can "leak." For example, cast iron pots leak iron.

FDA researchers claim, however, that the amount of material that leaks from the pots and pans into the food is not enough to cause any harm.

The levels of "leakage" are well within the FDA safety standards.

This is also true for chips of pot coatings.

If you chip a piece of the nonstick coating into your food, you don't need to throw out the food.

The chip will pass right through your digestive system without harming you at all.

So, the best choice of pots and pans really depends on personal preference.

Simple aspirin therapy helps prevent migraine headaches

Ugh! You can tell before it hits.

Bam! You dread it.

Pow! It won't be a regular headache. It will be a blinding, nauseating, incapacitating migraine.

Whew! Help might be closer than you think.

Migraine headaches and their causes are not well understood.

However, scientists suspect that one cause may be the platelets in the blood, says the *The Journal of the American Medical Association* (264,13:1711).

When a migraine occurs, the platelets get together and release a substance called serotonin. This causes the blood vessels to swell and produce the symptoms that make a migraine nearly unbearable.

The good news is that there is a way to prevent these platelets from clumping up.

The remedy is simple — take one aspirin every two days.

Studies show that this treatment helped people of all ages and all fitness levels. The aspirin cut migraines by 20 percent.

The trick is to begin this low dosage program before the migraine and then to continue the treatment during and after the attack to reduce your chances of having another migraine.

Some people are sensitive or allergic to aspirin. So you should check with your doctor before you start taking aspirin every other day.

Your doctor can recommend whether this is a safe and effective treatment for you.

Heart Problems

Ear crease could be early warning sign of fatal heart attack

A diagonal crease across your earlobe at a 45-degree downward angle toward your shoulder may be an early warning sign of a potentially fatal heart attack, according to reports in *Modern Medicine* (57,10:126) and *British Heart Journal* (611,4:361).

You might think we're pulling your, uh..., ears.

But, scientists have been studying the amazing ear-crease phenomenon since 1973 — with inconclusive results until this research report.

In the latest study, they found telltale ear creases in both fat and skinny people who died from sudden heart attacks, so weight wasn't a factor.

The common denominator was sudden death, often in people who apparently didn't know how sick they were.

In the current study, researchers randomly selected 303 people whose cause of death was unknown before autopsy.

They found diagonal ear creases in 72 percent of the deceased men and 67 percent of the deceased women.

Men with diagonal ear creases were 55 percent more likely to die of heart disease than men without ear creases.

The risk was even greater for non-diabetic women (1.74 times more likely to die of heart disease).

Interestingly, ear creases did not predict death from heart disease in diabetic women.

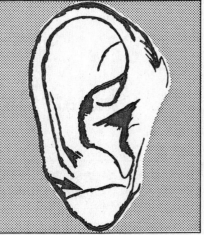

Those with ear creases generally don't get them until after age 50, the reports say.

Fatness apparently does not influence whether people have ear creases, researchers say, because both fat and thin people have them in roughly equal numbers.

However, people with heart disease seem to develop the creases, regardless of their age, they add.

The alarming thing was the link between ear creases and unexpected death.

Many people in this study had died suddenly from heart attacks, but had no history of heart disease, the researchers say.

In this group, earlobe creases alone were a greater predictor of sudden death from heart attack than known risk factors, such as previous heart disease, the studies report.

That fact has led researchers to speculate that some doctors may be missing severe heart disease cases among some middle-aged and elderly people. If that's the case, help yourself by checking your ears for diagonal creases.

If there is a crease, tell your doctor about the crease and about these studies.

The idea is to catch unsuspected heart disease so you can get appropriate treatment.

Graze your way to a healthier heart

Snacking during the day, sometimes called "grazing," may be better for your heart than eating three square meals a day, Canadian researchers report in *The New England Journal of Medicine* (321,14:929).

But that doesn't mean you can eat just potato chips and ice cream — or simply snack between meals.

To get the benefits, you must eat small, nutritious meals throughout the day, researchers say, and your calorie count must not increase.

Researchers believe snacking works by controlling the production of certain chemicals in the body.

Insulin, a hormone released by the pancreas, helps the body produce cholesterol. How much insulin the pancreas releases into the bloodstream depends on the size of the meals you eat.

Snackers may have lower cholesterol levels because they eat smaller amounts of food, and the pancreas produces less insulin in response.

Less insulin usually means less cholesterol.

Eating more meals throughout the day and adding more fiber to your diet may be keys to keeping your cholesterol levels under control.

During the study, seven men aged 31 to 51 ate three meals a day for two weeks or 17 snacks a day for two weeks and then switched to the other diet.

The snackers' insulin levels dropped by 28 percent during the study.

Their total cholesterol levels were 8.5 percent lower than men eating three meals a day.

Based on the results of this study, researchers believe that nutritious nibbling throughout the day may help you lower cholesterol levels and fight heart disease.

Add fish to your diet to help prevent fatal heart attacks

Eating fish at least twice a week might prolong your life, according to a new study in *The Lancet* (2,8666:757).

Even people with advanced heart disease could benefit, the two-year study suggests.

During a two-year study, 2,000 men who had suffered their first heart attacks received advice about fat, fish and fiber intake.

Those men who ate fatty fish — such as mackerel, herring, salmon and trout — or took fish oil supplements reduced their chances of dying from another heart attack by nearly one-third.

Those in the less-fat group had no added benefits, while those who ate more fiber actually showed a slight increase in fatal attacks.

Although eating fish didn't cut the number of new heart attacks, it seemed to cut the number of fatal attacks, the study indicates.

Researchers believe fish oil helps prevent clogged arteries, though it may take as long as two years to see any positive effects.

They plan more long-term studies.

Estrogen therapy fights heart disease?

Should women take estrogen replacements after menopause? Some experts believe they should because estrogen replacement therapy helps reduce a woman's risk of heart disease, says a recent report in *The Western Journal of Medicine* (152,4:408).

Pre-menopausal women have a lower rate of heart disease than men. Apparently, estrogen helps decrease total cholesterol levels and LDL ("bad" cholesterol) levels in the blood.

But estrogen increases HDL ("good" cholesterol) levels. In effect, the estrogen protects women from heart disease.

However, after menopause, women lose this advantage because they stop producing estrogen. When a woman produces less estrogen because of the onset of menopause or because of a surgical removal of her ovaries, her body no longer fights cholesterol build-up naturally. Obviously, this places her at a greater risk for heart disease. This causes a woman's risk of heart disease to increase at the same rate as a man's.

However, a woman can continue to benefit from the positive effects of estrogen if she replaces the estrogen that her body no longer produces.

According to a study reported in *Medical World News* (31,9:10), women who used estrogen replacement therapy were 40 percent less likely to die of heart attack than nonusers. Estrogen users also had a 50 percent lower risk of stroke than nonusers.

Yet estrogen replacement therapy is not for everyone. Women who still have a uterus must be especially careful.

Because of a risk of cancer and other diseases, these women must take progestin replacements along with the estrogen replacements.

The only problem is that progestin has the *opposite* effect on blood cholesterol levels than the estrogen does. Progestin raises the LDL levels and lowers the HDL levels, which increases the risk of heart disease.

However, some researchers have recently reported that even a small positive effect of estrogen replacement therapy would outweigh any increased risk of death from endometrial or breast cancer, according to a report in *Geriatrics* (45,5:84).

These researchers report that a 50-year-old white American woman has a 31 percent risk of developing heart disease and only a nine percent risk of breast cancer and a three percent risk of endometrial cancer. Since a very high number of women die from heart disease, these studies suggest that all women should consider estrogen therapy unless they have other risk factors.

The combined effects of progestin and estrogen therapies on the blood cholesterol depends on the kind of progestin used. Some forms of progestin do not affect the blood as much as other forms.

Your doctor can recommend which type of progestin and estrogen replacement therapies to use to obtain the best results and the greatest protection from heart problems.

Magnesium cuts risk of heart disease

Good news: if the drinking water in your area is considered "hard," that could be good news for your health! Hard water is rich in magnesium, and magnesium is a mineral that helps your nerves and muscles function properly.

Better news: scientists now realize that magnesium also plays a beneficial role in preventing heart disease. A new study described in *Science News* (137,14:214) suggests that magnesium teams up with a low-cholesterol diet to discourage atherosclerosis, or the build-up of fat deposits on the walls of coronary arteries.

Researchers believe that a good supply of magnesium in your diet discourages the production of cells that form the fatty deposits on artery walls.

Scientists also suggest that a diet that is too low in magnesium can cause your body to draw magnesium from your muscles. This reduces the amount of magnesium in the muscles that is necessary to keep the muscles working properly.

Unfortunately, magnesium alone will not prevent or cure atherosclerosis. Eating a low-cholesterol diet is still your best protection against this form of heart disease. However, you can strengthen your defenses by including high-magnesium foods in your menus.

Boost your body's supply of magnesium by eating more green vegetables, nuts, whole grains and shellfish — all good natural sources of this essential mineral. And as you protect your heart, you will also help your other muscles function smoothly.

Remember, check with your doctor before using vitamin supplements to increase your supply of magnesium.

Your heart's desire

Rest is no longer the best treatment for people who have had chronic heart failure. Doctors are now encouraging heart patients to exercise.

In a recent study, stable chronic heart failure patients who rode an exercise bike for 20 minutes, five days a week, showed improvement in exercise tolerance, peak oxygen use, heart rate and in symptoms of breathlessness, fatigue and general well-being, says a digest report in *Medical Abstracts* (10,2:3).

People who have had heart failure should talk to their doctor about the benefits of exercise. Your doctor can help plan an exercise program designed especially to meet your needs.

Bigger isn't better

The old saying "he has a big heart" may have more meaning than it once did.

Scientists have found that an enlarged heart may be hazardous to your health and could result in sudden death, even when other heart disease is absent.

This condition is known as left ventricular hypertrophy (LVH) and is often a result of years of high blood pressure, says a report in the *Cardiovascular Research Report* (34:2).

Taking measures to prevent or to lower high blood pressure decreases the risk of developing LVH.

'Miracle' clove reduces rates of heart attacks

For a long time, it seemed that garlic was popular with everybody except vampires and scientists.

For centuries, garlic has enjoyed great fame and popularity as a "miracle, cure-all" clove.

But scientists and researchers often dismissed the subject as simply another example of "primitive" folklore. Until now, that is.

Now, researchers are beginning to investigate the actual "powers" of garlic, and they like what they're finding.

One possible benefit of garlic compounds may be their anti-cancer effects.

Apparently, garlic increases the body's ability to remove substances in the blood that trigger cancer, says a recent study in *Preventive Medicine* (19,3: 346)

Garlic actually seems to "clean" the blood.

So, eating more garlic results in much lower rates of cancer, says the report.

For example, people in regions of China where average garlic consumption is high (a little less than one ounce per day) have lower rates of stomach cancer than people in the regions where the garlic intake is low.

Garlic also seems to reduce the rates of heart attacks.

Garlic eaters had 32 percent fewer second heart attacks and 45 percent fewer deaths from heart attacks than non-garlic eaters, reports the Sept. 8, 1990 issue of *Science News* (138,10:157).

Garlic also might interfere with the body's bad habit of over-producing cholesterol and other blood-clotting agents that contribute to heart disease, says *Science News*.

The moral of the story? Add an extra bit of garlic to your diet. It may be bad for your breath, but it could help save your life!

Olive oil gives double-barreled protection for your heart

Calling all cooks! Olive oil is good for more than tasty salads!

Studies show that olive oil provides double-barreled protection for your heart, reports the Oct. 4, 1990 *Medical Tribune* (31,20:15).

Olive oil is rich in monounsaturated fatty acids, and these fatty acids can have two positive effects on your health.

1. Lowers cholesterol. Your doctor has been telling you to avoid saturated and hydrogenated fats (usually hardened fats, such as cooking lard) because they can raise your cholesterol. However, olive oil is rich in unsaturated fats that can actually lower your LDL cholesterol level. (LDL cholesterol is the "bad" cholesterol.)

2. Reduces risk of atherosclerosis. This disease begins as "scratches" on the inside of your arteries. This is similar to rubbing coarse sandpaper on the inside of a plastic pipe. These "scratches" are a good place for cholesterol to attach and build up.

The scratches can be caused by a chemical change (oxidation) in the LDL cholesterol in your blood. The olive oil helps keep the chemical change in the LDL from happening. This reduces the chances of "scratches" forming and lowers your risk of heart disease.

So, stock your kitchen with olive oil. It's great in your salads, and it helps you protect a healthy heart!

If your spouse smokes, beware of heart disease

You're a nonsmoker, so you think you're safe from cardiovascular problems that are caused by smoking. But you could be mistaken, especially if your spouse smokes.

A recent study compared the number of cases of cardiovascular disease among nonsmoking women who were married to smokers with the number of cases among nonsmoking women whose husbands did not smoke.

The study revealed that women whose husbands smoked were 1.5 times more likely to die of cardiovascular disease than the women married to nonsmokers, says the *American Family Physician* (42,4:1080).

The passive smoke from your spouse's cigarette is dangerous to both of you. That is a good reason to encourage your spouse to quit smoking — it will help both of you avoid cardiovascular disease.

Nutrition

National Research Council updates RDA values

The labels on your cereal boxes and vitamin-mineral supplements probably are out of date.

That's because the familiar Recommended Daily Allowances (RDAs) published by the National Research Council have been changed.

These are the first such changes in nearly a decade.

In the new guidelines, published at the end of 1989, nutritionists give their estimates of healthy amounts of 11 vitamins and seven minerals needed for several age groups of males and females.

The new list adds recommended daily intakes of vitamin K and selenium.

Scientists warn that smokers need more vitamin C than anybody else, according to *Medical Tribune* (30,30:8).

Tobacco users need 100 milligrams of vitamin C a day, nearly twice as much as nonsmokers, according to the revised guidelines.

The RDA for nonsmokers of all ages remains at 60 milligrams, same as the old RDA chart.

Besides those three changes, the other revisions actually are reductions. Here are the major changes:

Vitamin K—The new RDA is 80 micrograms (abbreviated either "µg" or "mcg") for adult males over age 25, and 65 micrograms for adult females over age 25.

A microgram is one-millionth of a gram and equals one-thousandth of a milligram.

Vitamin C—100 milligrams for male and female smokers; 60 milligrams for everybody else.

Vitamin A—Unchanged at 1000 micrograms (equal to one milligram) for men and children.

It remains the same for women of all ages—800 micrograms—except for mothers who have just given birth and are producing milk (lactating). For them, the RDA is 1200 to 1300 micrograms.

The panel reduced the RDA for pregnant women from 1000 micrograms down to 800.

Folate — one of the family of B vitamins, the new RDA is reduced from 400 micrograms for both men and women to 200 micrograms for men and 180 micrograms for women.

By the way, folate is the same thing as folic acid and folacin.

Vitamin B6 — The new RDA is 2 milligrams for men and 1.6 milligrams for women.

That's reduced from 2.2 for men and 2 for women.

Vitamin B12 — Reduced from 3 micrograms to 2 micrograms for adult men and women.

Selenium—The new RDA is 70 micrograms for males over 25, and 55 micrograms for females over 25.

Calcium — Stays at 800 milligrams for adult men and women, including the elderly.

The change is for young women. The recommended level of 1200 milligrams is extended from teenagers through young women up to age 24.

The idea is that more calcium at an early age will help prevent crippling osteoporosis later in women's lives.

Iron — Remains at 10 milligrams for adult men and women after menopause, but is reduced from 18 milligrams to 15 for adolescent girls and adult women before menopause, according to the *Tribune* report.

Magnesium — Stays at 350 milligrams for men, but is cut for women from 300 to 280 milligrams, according to *Medical World News* (30,22:28).

Zinc — For adult women, reduced from 15 milligrams to 12. Remains at 15 milligrams for adult men.

Protein — For pregnant women, reduced from an extra 30 grams daily to an extra 10 grams per day.

In other words, instead of an expectant mother eating around an extra ounce of protein each day, the new recommendation calls for her to eat about an additional one-third ounce of protein daily.

The panel of nutritionists cut several RDAs, sometimes as much as one-half.

That's because new research indicates the body either stores more of these nutrients than was previously thought, or needs less to stay healthy, says Richard J. Havel at the University of California, San Francisco.

Havel was chairman of the panel that made the RDA changes.

Low-fat diet helps strengthen immune system

Are people who eat high-fat diets more likely to become ill?

Yes, say University of Massachusetts researchers in *The American Journal of Clinical Nutrition* (50,4:861).

A low-fat diet, combined with regular exercise, can help you build up your resistance against illness and disease, they add.

They studied 17 healthy, male nonsmokers 21 to 39 years old

who were not overweight.

After analyzing their diets, researchers advised them how to eat less fat.

After eating a low-fat diet for three months, the men were found to have built up a large supply of natural killer cells.

Natural killer cells form an important part of the body's immune system.

These specialized "warrior" cells attack and kill cancer and tumor cells.

In addition to improving immunity, the low-fat diet also helped the men control their weight. They ate fewer calories and exercised regularly.

Those two factors directly affect the build-up of killer cells, researchers say.

Scientists have known for some time that poor diet directly affects our ability to fight disease.

Some researchers suggest that diseases such as cancer may be linked to a "defective immune system."

In everyday terms, "defective immune system" means the same thing as lowered resistance.

The Massachusetts researchers are quick to point out that their study was small, not large enough to prove anything.

In addition, they say, a low-fat diet affects only natural killer cells, not the entire immune system.

Larger studies are needed to see whether women, cancer patients and the elderly would gain immunity from low-fat diets.

Fish oil may help prevent the development of gallstones

Fish oil not only helps reduce heart-disease risk by lowering cholesterol, but it may also help prevent gallstones, according to researchers at the Johns Hopkins University School of Medicine and reported in *Science News* (135:21:332).

Gallstones — actually, cholesterol "crystals" — form in the gallbladder, a pouch located near the liver. A substance known as bile flows from the liver through the bile duct to the gallbladder, where it is stored and used for digestion. If gallstones lodge in the bile duct, surgery is sometimes needed.

A main "ingredient" of bile is liquid cholesterol.

Researchers don't know how liquid cholesterol hardens into gallstones, but they believe that omega-3 fatty acids found in fish oil halt the process.

Researchers recently tested their theory on prairie dogs. They fed 16 animals high-cholesterol diets; half were given fish-oil supplements.

After two weeks, researchers removed the animals' gallbladders.

The eight animals given fish oil had no gallstones; the other eight did.

Researchers are hopeful humans will show the same results. They plan more studies.

Fish oil is not just a passing fad

It's in the news again, but it's not just a passing fad.

Omega-3 fish oil has definite health benefits for people of all ages, agreed more than 300 researchers at a recent health conference in Washington.

Studies indicate that men who eat two or three helpings of fish a week are 40 percent less likely to die of heart attacks than men who eat no fish, says a report in *The Atlanta Journal* (108,22).

"It is quite apparent that fish had a protective effect against coronary heart disease, as well as against cardiovascular death and death from all causes," says Dr. Therese Dolecek, a nutrition epidemiologist at the Bowman Gray School of Medicine in Winston-Salem, North Carolina.

Other researchers at the conference praised the benefits of omega-3, not only for its role in preventing and treating heart disease, but also for its apparent beneficial effects on cancer, diabetes and psoriasis.

Studies show that omega-3 in infant formula appears to improve vision in premature infants, slows the buildup of platelets and other substances such as cholesterol on blood vessel walls, and helps reduce problems with irregular heart rhythms.

Omega-3 may also help rheumatoid arthritis sufferers.

Fish oil — how much is enough?

About three grams a day, or a little under one ounce a week, of omega-3 fatty acids—commonly known as "fish oil"—is the best dose size for cutting levels of fat in the blood, say researchers in *The American Journal of Clinical Nutrition* (52,1:120).

In a Dutch study, researchers at Amsterdam's Free University Hospital tested the effects of four different dosages of omega-3 oils on several types of cholesterol and triglycerides, as well as on the germ-killing power of white blood cells.

The doses tested ranged from zero to six grams a day. It takes 28 grams to make one ounce.

Triglycerides are a form of fat carried by the blood. Scientists consider high levels of triglycerides to be a risk factor for heart disease.

They found that fish oil even in small doses reduces triglycerides and raises the concentration of HDL ("good") cholesterol.

The effect was dose-dependent, meaning that the more fish oil taken by the volunteers, the more the benefits.

Up to a point, that is. Above three grams of fish oil per day, the body seems to be unable to use the extra fatty acids in a beneficial way.

Feeding the volunteers six grams per day had no more effect than giving them three grams a day, the researchers report.

Fish oil can decrease the blood's ability to form clots. In addition, some people report heartburn and belching as side-effects of taking fish oil capsules.

Check with your doctor before taking any omega-3 supplements.

A natural way to get the benefits of omega-3 is to eat cold-water fish two or three times a week, suggest many nutritionists.

Eat less protein to prevent further kidney damage

A low-protein diet can reduce the chances of further kidney damage for diabetics and other people with kidney diseases, researchers report in *The Lancet* (2,8677:1411).

For years doctors have advised diabetics to eat the same amount of protein as healthy people.

But now they're saying that too much protein could stimulate more blood flow into the kidneys, making them work harder. This extra strain on the kidneys could be dangerous.

You have a better chance of avoiding kidney damage if you follow a low-protein diet in the early stages of a kidney disease, researchers say.

Low-protein diets cannot stop kidney damage in the late or final stages of a serious kidney disease, they add.

In a British study of 19 people in various stages of kidney disease, a low-protein diet reduced stress on the kidneys and slowed kidney damage.

Similarly, an 18-month Australian study of 64 diabetics showed that restricting protein intake delays kidney damage.

Half of the group ate their regular diet, while the other half ate a protein-restricted diet.

Nine of 33 people on the regular diet developed kidney failure, compared with only two of 31 people on the protein-restricted diet.

Although a low-protein diet seems to be the best way to protect kidneys from further damage, be very careful about changing your diet.

A drastic change may do more harm than good.

Your doctor or nutritionist can help you plan a safe and healthy diet to suit your nutritional needs and give you the best possible results.

Eat less to live longer

Saying "no thanks" to seconds at the dinner table may actually help prolong your life, Texas researchers report in *Geriatrics* (44:12,87).

Reducing calories prolonged the lives of healthy rats in their study, but did not stunt growth, researchers said. Even animals with heart and kidney problems lived longer and developed tumors later in life than rats on unrestricted diets.

The rats on restricted diets lived longer than those who ate freely, researchers said.

Other benefits of a disciplined diet include healthier bones and improved immunity, they added.

Would humans reap similar benefits? Scientists have known for some time that diet, growth and aging are related, but animal studies such as this are the first step in understanding how diet may prolong human life.

Researchers have several theories. This study suggests that digesting three well-balanced meals a day constitutes an "eight-hour workday" for your body. Eating more than you need means your cells must work overtime to digest the extra food.

"Tired" cells weaken with age and can't fight disease and illness effectively. In a nutshell, the less you eat, the less work for your body.

What you eat may also be a significant factor in prolonging life, researchers said. Chemicals in certain foods cause a "red alert" in your body, meaning that it must work double-overtime to digest them.

Further studies will look at what foods cause this response in the body.

In the meantime, eating less seems to have many more positive benefits than always eating until you're stuffed.

Low-fat diet fights heart disease

Lower your cholesterol without cutting back on calories? Eat meat, and lower harmful LDL cholesterol at the same time? It sounds improbable, but the results of a recent study suggest that it is possible, even for people with heart disease.

According to a study in *The Wall Street Journal* (3/23/90), one way to fight heart disease is with simple, effective changes in your diet. To demonstrate this, researchers watched a group of men with proven coronary heart disease over a two-year period.

The men in the study didn't cut back on the number of calories they ate, and they didn't lose weight. Instead, they lowered the amount of fat in their diets by substituting protein calories for fat calories.

By changing the kinds of foods they ate, these men reduced the amount of fat in their diet to an average of 27.5 percent of their total calorie intake. As a result, no new fat deposits formed on the walls of their coronary arteries, and their blood levels of LDL cholesterol went down.

On the other hand, the men who allowed their fat intake to exceed 30 percent of their total calories developed new fatty deposits on the walls of their arteries, risking more heart trouble in the future.

These dramatic results should encourage people, especially those with coronary heart disease, to change their diets to help fight heart disease. As a goal, the National Cholesterol Education program recommends that you lower your fat calories to less than 30 percent of your total caloric intake. To start with, choose lean meats instead of fatty meats and use low-fat dairy products instead of those with a high-fat content.

Switching to low-fat foods may not seem that important on a daily basis, but this simple change can make a big difference to your heart.

Oat bran extract

Lower your blood cholesterol level by eating ice cream!

A fantasy, you say?

U.S. Department of Agriculture scientists say they have come up with a new process that extracts the fat-fighting part of oat bran and turns it into a creamy substance that could be used to replace many kinds of fats in foods, including ice cream.

Called oatrim, the white, tasteless flour is loaded with beta-glucans, the part of oat bran that researchers believe lowers cholesterol levels. Researchers treat oat bran with enzymes to produce either a flour or a powder.

In animal tests, oatrim slashed cholesterol by 18 percent. Even better, it hits hardest at LDL cholesterol, the "bad" form, while it seems to slightly increase HDL or "good" cholesterol, says a report in *The Wall Street Journal* (215,79:B1).

Adding about an ounce of oatrim to an instant breakfast drink gives you more cholesterol-lowering beta-glucans than three ounces of pure oat bran, the report says.

Raw vegetables help guard against cholesterol build-up

Four ounces of raw broccoli contains twice as much vitamin C as four ounces of orange juice made from frozen concentrate.

If the broccoli is really fresh — just-picked broccoli has a bluish-green color — it contains nearly 40 percent more than stalks that have been in the store for a few days.

But freeze the broccoli, or steam it, blanch it, boil it, or otherwise cook it in any way, and it loses half its vitamin C content, says a report in *Science News* (137,23:367).

Some research indicates that vitamin C serves as a powerful guard against build-ups of cholesterol on artery walls.

That protects against hardening of the arteries and lowers the risks of heart attacks and strokes.

Other protective substances in broccoli, cabbage and related cruciferous vegetables also lose their potency when hit by cooking heat.

Cooked vegetables are good for you, the report reaffirms.

But the best deal is to eat veggies raw and as fresh as you can get them.

"It" has long-term benefits

"It" can keep you out of the hospital. "It" can save your life.

If you knew what "it" was, would you do "it"?

"It" is very simple — a balanced diet.

A study of 59 elderly people who were hospitalized for a break within the hip joint shows important results — a poor diet can demand a high price.

A poor diet can cause calcium to leave the bones and enter the bloodstream, weaken the bones and make them more likely to break during a fall.

According to a report in *The Lancet* (335,8696:1013), poor nutrition can also weaken muscles, reduce our sense of balance and reaction time and increase the chance of falling while just walking around.

Also, muscles that do not receive proper nutrition are less able to protect us when we fall.

These combined problems which stem from poor nutrition can increase your chances of being hospitalized after a fall. But, there are benefits of eating a balanced diet and getting good nutrition.

A properly balanced diet can increase muscle strength, coordination and reaction time while building stronger bones. These combined benefits of good nutrition can work together to keep you out of the hospital.

There are other benefits, too. If you are hospitalized, you will be less likely to develop bedsores. People who are well nourished get well quicker than poorly nourished people.

They also have fewer infections, such as pneumonia. The most important difference is that people are more likely to live after a serious hospitalization if they are well nourished.

What should you do now? Make sure you are receiving proper nutrition. If you are not sure, see your doctor for advice.

Eat a balanced diet to decrease your chances of being hospitalized, to decrease your recovery time if hospitalization is necessary and to live longer and healthier.

Officials hope for 20 percent reduction in heart disease

Even healthy adults should skip the cheeseburger and fries for lunch. The fat content of that one meal just might be more than double your recommended daily allowance of fat.

According to the *Medical Tribune* (31,7:4), the government is now recommending dietary changes intended to reduce the average American's cholesterol by 10 percent.

Officials of the National Cholesterol Education Program (NCEP) hope for a 20 percent reduction in coronary heart disease over the next five to ten years if their suggestions for eating patterns are taken seriously.

The NCEP's lower-fat diet consists of leaner meats, lower-fat dairy products, more fruits and vegetables, beans, and whole-grain products. The ultimate goal is to keep your total cholesterol intake to less than 300 milligrams daily and your daily fat intake to less than 30 percent of the daily caloric intake.

Until recently, only people with existing cholesterol problems were asked to stick to dietary changes aimed at lowering their risk of heart disease. But now, due to the benefits of preventive medicine, everyone can put a healthy distance between themselves and heart attack.

Psyllium more effective than oat bran?

Many people today rely on oat bran and other whole grains to help lower cholesterol and add fiber to their diet. But scientists may have discovered an even more effective source of soluble fiber.

According to *The Wall Street Journal* (4/3/90), cereals containing the grain psyllium are more effective than oat bran and other fibers at lowering blood cholesterol.

Psyllium is not a new discovery, but you might not recognize it by that name. You may know it as the grain called flea wort.

And you may already be familiar with psyllium in another form. Procter & Gamble has used it for years in the laxative Metamucil.

Three studies backed by the Kellogg Company measured psyllium's effectiveness in reducing cholesterol levels of people already on a low-cholesterol diet. The test results suggested that psyllium is more effective than oat bran at lowering cholesterol.

These studies concluded that psyllium cereals are safe to eat. However, after you add psyllium-containing cereals to your diet, you may begin to notice some minor side effects, especially if you are not used to eating high-fiber cereals.

A sudden increase in fiber consumption can cause gas, bloating and cramping. So, begin with a small amount of psyllium-enriched cereal to avoid unnecessary side effects.

Whether you know psyllium as the grain flea wort or simply as an addition to your breakfast cereal, it can provide another valuable way to lower your cholesterol and add fiber to your diet.

"Stress" causes cancer?

Stress is usually caused by hectic schedules, rush hour traffic and other obviously stressful situations.

But you may be creating the most dangerous kind of stress at your supper table!

Recent studies show that you may be putting dangerous stress on your body by eating certain foods, not eating the right proportion of one food to another food, and by eating the wrong kinds of foods.

According to a report in the *Journal of the National Cancer*

Institute (82,6: 491), the hidden stress caused by this "stress diet" may actually encourage cancer to begin growing in your intestines.

What is a "stress diet"? Unfortunately, it is typical of the diet of most people in the United States. The "stress diet" has four problem areas that you should watch for.

1. Not enough calcium. Some sources recommend up to 1500 milligrams per day, but the average American only gets 500 to 600 milligrams per day.

To increase your daily calcium intake, eat more foods that contain calcium, such as milk, cheese, yogurt and molasses. You may also consider taking calcium supplements.

2. Not enough vitamin D. Vitamin D helps your body absorb and use calcium. So a vitamin D deficiency also can cause a calcium deficiency.

Also, studies show that if you get enough vitamin D, you are less likely to get colon cancer. Vitamin D is found in egg yolks, organ meats and bone meal.

You also can get vitamin D by spending a few minutes each day in the sunlight. Sunlight produces vitamin D naturally in the body.

3. Too much phosphorus in relation to calcium. You need equal amounts of phosphorus and calcium in your diet.

The Recommended Daily Allowance (RDA) for phosphorus and calcium is 800 milligrams for each.

Many Americans get 1500 milligrams of phosphorus or more per day and only 500 to 600 milligrams of calcium per day.

Too much phosphorus can keep your body from using the calcium it needs.

4. Too much fat. Most people in the U.S. get about 40 percent of their calories from fat. Animal fats and some polyunsaturated vegetable oils (such as corn oil) contain fats which promote the development of cancer.

Scientists recommend that you decrease your intake of red meats and polyunsaturated vegetable oils. Then increase your intake of "good" fat such as safflower, sunflower, soy and canoli oils.

If your diet contains one or more of these four "stress" factors, you may be creating extra hidden stress in your body that could eventually lead to colon cancer. Eliminating the "stress" from your diet could decrease your risk of cancer.

But remember, you should discuss any drastic changes in your diet with your doctor to guarantee your best health.

Soup seasoning is good food

Maybe you have always used a single basil leaf to season your homemade soups.

Now scientists say that basil is good for more than just a seasoning for your homemade vegetable soup.

According to a digest in *HerbalGram* (20:23), the use of basil might help you increase your body's physical endurance and resistance to stress and disease.

Unsaturated fats: how do you know if they are 'good' or 'bad'?

Forget saturated and unsaturated fats.

From now on, think of fats this way: there's good fat and there's bad fat.

But, you argue, my doctor has been stressing the importance of eating unsaturated fats and steering clear of saturated fats.

Well, now there's a new twist to the story, says this week's *The New England Journal of Medicine* (323,7:439).

Usually, unsaturated fats are better for you than saturated fats. But now you need to watch which kinds of unsaturated fats you eat.

The kinds of unsaturated fats that you now need to avoid are known as "trans" fatty acids — the "bad" fats. These trans fatty acids are formed by a process called "hydrogenation."

During the hydrogenation process, regular unsaturated fatty acids ("good" fats) are changed into a different form. Instead of being in liquid form at room temperature, they are changed into solid form. (This is kind of like ice and water — the same substance in two different forms.)

The new, solid form of these unsaturated fatty acids is referred to as "trans" or "hydrogenated," and they are used in baking products such as margarines and shortenings.

So, you say, . . .what's the problem?

Well, here's the clincher.

The effect that these "bad" unsaturated fatty acids have on your cholesterol level is worse than the effect of saturated fatty acids.

Trans fatty acids ("bad" fats) raise levels of LDL serum cholesterol ("bad" cholesterol) and lower the levels of HDL serum cholesterol ("good" cholesterol).

This produces the highest — and the unhealthiest — ratio of total cholesterol to HDL cholesterol. And that high ratio is a huge risk factor for coronary heart disease.

In the typical American diet, two to four percent of the calories come from these dangerous "bad" fatty acids.

Researchers suggest that it would be a good idea for people who have an increased risk of atherosclerosis to avoid a high intake of "bad" fatty acids.

One way to avoid a high intake of "bad" fatty acids is to read labels very carefully.

Look for the difference in fats that have been "partially hydrogenated" and those that have been "completely hydrogenated."

The partially hydrogenated fats are the "trans" fatty acids — avoid them.

Regular unsaturated fatty acids ("good" fats) that haven't been hydrogenated at all are your best bet.

Try to use liquid vegetable oils instead of hardened vegetable oils.

And, as always, try to keep your total fat intake below 30 percent of your daily intake of calories.

Soybean extract reverses liver disease

Years of heavy alcohol consumption often result in severe liver damage, cirrhosis of the liver. Until now, cirrhosis has been untreatable.

But 12 hard-drinking baboons in New York might point the way to preventing and even reversing the deadly disease, according to the Dec. 1, 1990 *Science News* (138,22:340).

Many of the baboons in the New York study probably felt no pain. After all, doctors were feeding the ape-like animals the alcohol equivalent of eight cans of beer a day.

Along with the alcohol, some animals received a diet supplemented daily with three tablespoons of soybean lecithin. Others ate just regular baboon foods, without the lecithin.

Most of those fed alcohol without lecithin developed severe scarring of the liver, including two cases of cirrhosis.

But the eight-beers-a-day group that got the daily lecithin

developed almost no scarring, even after eight years of hard drinking, the *SN* report says.

To clinch the case for lecithin, researchers kept on feeding alcohol to three of the baboons but withheld all lecithin. Within two years, all three animals had developed cirrhosis.

Another researcher reported that lecithin apparently heals liver tissue scarred by alcohol. That might mean a reversal of early cirrhosis damage, the report says.

Animal tests don't always translate into human benefits. Researchers caution that people who drink too much alcohol should cut back or stop drinking, rather than seeking some "magic pill" to allow them to continue their substance abuse.

Lecithin is a natural part of many foods. It is a major dietary source of the nutrient choline. Natural sources of lecithin include soybeans, lentils, beans, peas, rice, cauliflower, eggs, cabbage and calves' liver. It's also used as an emulsifying agent in prepared foods like mayonnaise and chocolates.

Lecithin has been used as an experimental treatment for Alzheimer's disease without much success. Among its unproven benefits are improved memory and lowered cholesterol levels.

There is no official Recommended Dietary Allowance (RDA) for lecithin, although many health food stores sell it in tablet, powder and liquid forms. Taking too much lecithin can result in a fishy body odor.

If you suffer from cirrhosis, check with your doctor before taking lecithin or supplements of any kind.

Osteoporosis

Too much salt causes body to lose calcium

Too much salt in the diet may increase a woman's chances of suffering osteoporosis after menopause, Canadian researchers report in *The American Journal of Clinical Nutrition* (50,5:1088).

They studied 17 women aged 52 to 72 who ate their usual diet and were then given salt supplements.

Excess salt causes the body to rid itself of calcium through urination, researchers say. Many postmenopausal women do not get enough calcium to begin with, they add.

If salt intake is low, women susceptible to osteoporosis might need less calcium after menopause, a New Zealand team of researchers concludes in the *British Medical Journal* (299,6703:834).

Thus, if you eat less salt, you might enjoy better bone health, the study suggests.

Ten women over age 65 volunteered for the study. They alternated their regular diet with low-salt and high-salt diets for periods of 10 days.

Women on the low-salt diet had the least loss of calcium,

followed by the regular diet and high-salt diet groups.

Osteoporosis is a crippling bone disease that strikes mostly among women over 50.

Osteoporosis affects men as well as women

Osteoporosis — the brittle-bone disease — is non-discriminatory after all, affecting both women and men, new research suggests.

Latest finding: men in later life lose about 2.3 percent of spinal bone every year, reports a study in *Annals of Internal Medicine* (112:1:29).

Men from age 30 on lose about 1 percent per year of bone mass in the wrists and hands, the study says.

The rate of bone loss in the hands and wrists gets worse as men get older, the study says.

Until now, most researchers thought osteoporosis affected mainly women past menopause.

For that reason, nutritionists recently boosted the Recommended Dietary Allowance (RDA) of calcium for younger women, believing more calcium at a younger age may help prevent brittle bones in later years.

Now, they may have to rethink the RDA for younger men as well.

Unfortunately, the study also suggested that taking calcium supplements later in life seemed not to stop or even to slow the rate of bone loss in men.

"We found a substantial rate of bone loss, despite a generous calcium intake," the study reports.

Osteoporosis causes the stooped posture and distinctive "dowager's hump" in elderly women.

It's also responsible for many of the hip, leg and arm fractures suffered by many older people, the report says.

Vitamin D helps fight crippling bone loss

If you have passed menopause and want to protect yourself from osteoporosis, be careful not to neglect your vitamin D. According to a report in *The New England Journal of Medicine* (321,26:1777), vitamin D is an important weapon in fighting crippling bone loss.

Without proper amounts of vitamin D, your body cannot regulate the level of parathyroid hormones that it makes. Parathyroid hormones can speed up bone loss by interfering with the body's absorption of calcium.

It's true that calcium is a major building block of strong bones, but you can't eat enough foods rich in calcium to make up for a diet low in vitamin D. When vitamin D levels drop, too many parathyroid hormones are produced.

When this happens, the body loses its ability to use the extra calcium.

In other words, you may be eating a lot of calcium, but your body can't use it because you don't have enough vitamin D.

Unless vitamin D levels are increased, you still run the risk of harmful bone loss, even with added calcium.

Researchers stress the importance of getting enough vitamin D in the diet, especially when exposure to sunlight is limited.

Your body produces vitamin D naturally in sunlight, enabling the body to keep parathyroid hormones below dangerous levels.

Vitamin D supplements during winter months help maintain hormone levels that would ordinarily vary from summer to winter. Without the advantage of vitamin D supplements, many women experience seasonal bone loss.

The report also states there is no evidence that an intake of vitamin D sufficient to protect you in winter would be intolerable during warm-weather exposure to the sun.

Drug and vitamin therapy may reverse effects of osteoporosis

A combination of the drug etidronate, calcium and vitamin D, all taken by mouth, seems to reverse the effects of osteoporosis.

The seven-city study involved 423 women who were past menopause and had spinal fractures caused by osteoporosis, according to the report in *The New England Journal of Medicine* (323,2:73).

After two years, the group receiving etidronate recorded a 5 percent gain in dense, new bone in the spine. A group receiving only calcium and vitamin D lost bone mass. The number of new spinal fractures in the etidronate group was half that of the others.

An earlier study in Denmark also used the same combination and had about the same results, says the May 3, 1990 *NEJM* (322,18:1265).

Etidronate is a drug that suppresses formation of osteoclasts. Osteoclasts are scavenger cells whose job is to destroy old bone cells.

In osteoporosis, the bone-eating cells destroy more strong bone than the body can replace, leading to soft, porous bones and increased fractures, says *Science News* (138,2:22).

Fluoride fails to prevent osteoporosis

Thinner, weaker bones trouble many women in the years

after menopause. In other countries, doctors have widely recommended sodium fluoride as a treatment for this condition. But, according to the *Mayo Clinic Health Letter* (8,4:5), new bone growth stimulated by sodium fluoride is so weak that it actually fractures more easily.

The best way to strengthen your bones is to exercise regularly and eat a diet rich in calcium-containing foods like dark green vegetables, dairy products and canned salmon or sardines.

Smoking and drinking too much alcohol can also increase your risk of developing osteoporosis.

Ask your dentist about the risk of developing brittle-bone disease

Swedish researchers are urging dentists to be on the look-out for warning signs of osteoporosis.

Recent studies reported in the *British Medical Journal* (300, 6730:1024) have shown that the fewer teeth women have, the greater their chances of developing brittle-bone disease.

Women should ask their dentists to be alert for two warning signs — loss of teeth and gum disease (problems with the tissues around the teeth).

If these conditions are present, women should consult their doctors about osteoporosis risks.

Too much caffeine may increase your risk of brittle-bone disease

People who drink large amounts of caffeinated beverages, such as coffee and tea, may have an increased risk of osteoporosis, reports the Oct. 10, 1990 *Science News* (138,16:253).

Osteoporosis is the "brittle-bone disease" that causes many broken and fractured bones in the elderly.

Researchers suggest that people who drink two to three cups of caffeinated coffee daily, or five to six cups of caffeinated tea daily, have almost a 70 percent greater risk of osteoporosis than those people who do not drink caffeine.

And people who drink three to four cups of coffee daily or six to seven cups of tea daily seem to have an 82 percent increased risk of osteoporosis compared to people who do not drink caffeinated beverages.

Apparently, the caffeine prevents the digestive system from absorbing enough calcium from the diet, and caffeine increases the amount of calcium that is lost in the urine.

The decreased amount of calcium in the body can result in osteoporosis.

So, if you drink caffeinated drinks, make sure you keep the number of cups each day below a safe level.

Seasonal Affective Disorder

Beat SADness and depression with light therapy

You've got the blues. You're craving starches, gaining weight, sleeping longer. You crave sunshine and want to hibernate.

What's wrong?

You may have seasonal affective disorder, commonly called SAD, which affects 5 million Americans every year, according to a recent report in *Postgraduate Medicine* (86,5:309).

SAD — four times more common in men than women — is depression often triggered by winter's short, dark days.

A lack of sunshine apparently throws some people into deep depression, which usually lifts in spring.

SAD also can occur in summer but is most common in winter.

The report outlines the SAD symptoms.

Where you live may influence your chances of suffering winter depression, reports *Science News* (136,15:198).

In a survey of patients visiting doctor's offices in Florida, Maryland, New York and New Hampshire, only 1.4 percent of Floridians reported SAD symptoms, compared with nearly 10 percent of New Hampshire residents.

Florida's sunny climate may explain the difference, researchers said.

Another study showed that 9 percent of Alaskans suffer through winter depression.

You don't have to move south to beat winter depression.

A megadose of artificial light for one to two hours in the morning should do it, researchers report in *Postgraduate Medicine* (86,5:309).

You'll need a light box (which you can buy) that produces light five times brighter than office light.

You should read or work about three feet from the light source and "glance at the lights a few times each minute," the study says.

If you feel eye strain or headache, sit farther away from the box, the report says.

You should notice some improvement in your mood after four days, these researchers say.

After two weeks, you can reduce the exposure to two or three times a week but should continue the "treatment" until winter ends, the doctors say.

Obviously, check with your doctor before trying this technique yourself.

Take advantage of sunny winter days as well.

Light therapy readjusts your circadian rhythm, or 24-hour sleep-wake cycle. The circadian rhythm responds to light, telling the body when it's time to sleep and time to wake up.

The internal clock also regulates other functions, such as body temperature, which is highest at bedtime to protect the body from cold during sleep, according to a report in *Medical Tribune* (30,26:1).

During the winter when the days are short and often cloudy, your circadian rhythm may "fall behind," causing you to sleep as much as 16 hours a day.

A megadose of artificial light in the morning helps "jump start" your internal clock and readjust it to winter's dark days.

Researchers use light therapy to help not only SAD sufferers, but shift workers, frequent travelers suffering from jet lag and elderly people with sleep disturbances, according to the *Medical Tribune* report.

Although internal-clock changes occur naturally with aging, doctors often fight the process with sleeping medications rather than help patients adjust to the change.

Light therapy may also help elderly people with Alzheimer's disease, 60 percent of whom are sleepwalkers, according to the report.

Researchers are studying how Alzheimer's disease affects a person's sleep-wake cycle.

Are you SAD? Here's a list of symptoms

- A bout of severe depression at least once during your lifetime.
- Regularly occurring fall and winter depression; the depression disappears in spring.
- Increased appetite, weight gain and carbohydrate cravings.
- Excessive sleep.
- For women, more severe premenstrual symptoms.
- No other psychiatric disorder.
- No other events (change in job or marital or

financial status, for example) that would affect mood.

Skin Problems

Get relief from irritating dry skin problems

Are you bothered with dry, chapped or itching skin? If so, you're not alone.

Dry skin is one of the most common skin problems in people everywhere.

Nearly everyone over 70 years of age has dry skin, says a report in *U.S. Pharmacist* (15,1:20). And eight out of every 10 people over age 60 have dry skin between November and March.

Dry skin is caused when the skin loses water.

Often the skin loses its moisture due to very dry air inside heated or air-conditioned buildings.

The dry air causes the skin to lose water faster than the body can replace it.

Dry skin also can be caused by rubbing and scratching, especially from wool clothes.

Symptoms of dry skin include redness, roughness, itching, scaling and chapping.

Lips also can become cracked and irritated.

Many people believe that moisturizing lotions alone can put

the wet back into dry skin. So they apply lotions several times a day, but they still have dry skin.

Others think that dry skin can be treated with longer baths. So they take more baths, but they can't get rid of the dry skin.

However, the best treatment for dry skin is to **replace** the lost moisture and then **protect** the skin from losing more water, using the "soak-grease" method:

(1) Soak in water for 5-10 minutes.

(2) Gently blot the skin dry (do not rub).

(3) Then apply a thin coat of lotion, cream or oil.

Soaking in water replaces the lost water in the skin, and then the lotion prevents the moisture from leaving the skin.

Men and women with dry skin also should drink at least six to eight glasses of clear liquid, preferably water, each day to help fight dry skin.

This does not include caffeinated or alcoholic drinks, which may cause more water loss from the skin.

A humidifier or vaporizer adds moisture to the air at home or at work. This helps protect your skin from drying out.

If you try the soak-grease method, drink lots of liquids, use a humidifier, and still have dry skin, see your doctor.

Unexplained dry skin can be a side effect of a more serious illness like diabetes mellitus and should be discussed with your doctor.

Tips to relieve dry skin

■ Try to avoid rubbing or scratching your skin if it itches. If itching becomes unbearable, talk to your pharmacist or doctor.

■ Don't wear woolen or other rough clothing. If

you do wear these items, wear a cotton shirt, blouse, or garment underneath.

■ Cover your skin when outside in the winter, to protect it from the wind and chilling air.

■ Wear rubber gloves when washing dishes or other work that involves putting your hands or arms in soapy water.

■ Drink at least 6 to 8 glasses of water or clear liquid each day. Limit your intake of caffeinated or alcoholic drinks.

■ Don't apply cosmetics or perfumed products over areas of dry skin, or on other areas of your body that itch.

■ If your home heating system doesn't have a humidifier system built in, use portable vaporizers or humidifiers to help add moisture to the air. Your pharmacist can help you select suitable units.

■ Use warm, not hot, water for bathing and cleansing your skin. Don't use strong soaps or detergents, and don't add bubble bath to the water.

■ Use a soft cloth or sponge to cleanse your skin. Don't use rough cloth or brushes.

■ Following bathing, pat your skin dry; don't rub it with a towel. Then, apply a thin layer of lotion or oil.

■ Avoid frequent bathing. Don't take saunas or steam baths, and don't soak in hot tubs.

■ Be careful getting into or out of a tub if you have used bath oil in the water. The tub's surface may become slippery.

Source: *U.S. Pharmacist* (15,1:22)

Contact dermatitis: a touchy subject

When you get a rash that itches, burns and stings, chances are you have contact dermatitis. That means you are allergic or sensitive to something that has touched your skin. The key to curing it is to find the source of irritation, but that may be easier said than done.

Most contact dermatitis is caused by an allergic reaction. A chemical that irritates the skin either on the first exposure or after repeated contact can cause non-allergic contact dermatitis, too.

Although it is common, contact dermatitis is hard to diagnose because there are so many possible sources.

Nickel-based jewelry, detergents, dish-washing soaps, deodorants, cosmetics, hair-care products, and some rubber products . . . all of these can cause inflammation.

You can even develop contact dermatitis from breathing in an airborne pollutant.

To complicate the situation, you can actually have allergic and non-allergic reactions at the same time. Sometimes even the medicine you use for a skin infection will cause contact dermatitis, making your problems worse.

In the face of these odds, how can you go about finding relief from contact dermatitis?

Various non-prescription remedies will soothe your discomfort, but the best solution is to identify the source of irritation. If you can avoid it, your contact dermatitis will probably go away.

Notice where you are having the problem. If you suspect you know the source of the irritation, avoid it to see if your rash clears up.

If you cannot locate the source, or your dermatitis gets worse, contact your doctor for help.

Talk to your pharmacist about how to use the treatments for contact dermatitis safely. You may be able to get relief by using oral antihistamines, wet dressings and anti-itch baths such as colloidal oatmeal.

According to *U.S. Pharmacist* (15,5:13), hydrocortisone cream is the most effective remedy for contact dermatitis.

If you use a hydrocortisone remedy for seven days without getting relief from your rash, you should stop using hydrocortisone. Your problem could be more complicated, and you may need to see a dermatologist to get relief.

Although contact dermatitis is common and uncomfortable, it is usually not serious. However, occasionally it gets bad enough to force a person to change jobs to escape an irritant.

If you think you have contact dermatitis, the best remedy is to find the source and avoid it.

What's causing the itch ... from head to toe

U.S. Pharmacist (15,5:14) has compiled this list of common causes of contact dermatitis:

Head — hair-care products, cosmetics, medicated skin creams, plants, face creams, hair spray, nail polish, nickel earrings, perfume, earphones, telephone receivers, lipstick, lip salves, toothpastes, mouthwash, clothing, cologne and jewelry.

Body — clothing, dress shields, deodorant, depilatories, medicated skin creams, hand lotions, soaps and detergents, rubber gloves and rubber bands, plants, douches, tampons, "jock itch" medicine, contraceptives (creams, rubber diaphragms, condoms), and hemorrhoid products.

Feet — athlete's foot medicine, stockings, slippers, shoes and shower sandals.

A new twist to aspirin pain relief

"Take an aspirin and call me in the morning."

You've heard this phrase a hundred times. But now it has a new twist.

Instead of taking an aspirin by mouth, many researchers are telling people to crush an aspirin, mix it with body lotion, and apply it to their skin.

Applying this mixture to your skin seems to provide relief from the intense pain that often comes with shingles, a skin disease caused by a herpes virus, says a report in *Medical Tribune* (31,2:9). This is the same virus that causes chicken pox in children.

People suffering from pain caused by the virus have not been able to find anything to relieve the pain. Until now, that is.

Scientists suggest crushing one 325-milligram aspirin tablet and mixing it into two tablespoons of Vaseline Intensive Care Lotion, then applying it to the skin three to four times daily.

Apparently, the skin absorbs the aspirin very quickly and easily, so the aspirin gives quick relief from the pain.

Researchers report that a 67-year-old man with Parkinson's disease responded to the aspirin-lotion mixture almost immediately (within 15 minutes).

Before using the lotion, he had been having trouble sleeping due to severe pain in his left shoulder caused by the herpes virus.

After three weeks of applying the aspirin-lotion mixture, he was able to sleep peacefully through the night.

Avoid alcohol if you suffer from psoriasis

A high alcohol intake worsens psoriasis, Finnish researchers report in the *British Medical Journal* (300,6727:780).

For two years, they studied 429 men (144 with psoriasis and 285 with other skin diseases) aged 19 to 50 and asked them the following questions:

• Does drinking increase the risk of psoriasis?
• Does drinking worsen psoriasis?
• Does psoriasis increase drinking?

Participants filled out a questionnaire about their drinking habits the year before their skin disease developed and the year before they joined the study.

Psoriasis was not associated with any other factor, such as age, social class or marital status.

"Alcohol intake and frequency of intoxication were individually the only significant explaining variables," researchers said.

Also, psoriasis patients reported that their drinking had increased after the disease was diagnosed, and one third reported that alcohol seemed to worsen their psoriasis.

Those who had psoriasis on a greater portion of their body tended to drink more as well.

Those findings lead researchers to suggest that psoriasis "sustains" drinking in some patients.

Poisonous plants put the itch in summer

If you're heading for the great outdoors this season, chances are you're also heading for a patch of poison ivy, poison oak or poison sumac.

And whenever the oil from any part of these plants touches you, it can cause an allergic skin reaction that may be red, blistered and oozing, reports *U.S. Pharmacist* (15,5:86).

This rash breaks out gradually and itches intensely for 10 to 14 days. Most people are allergic to these plants, so your best protection is to know what they look like and avoid touching them.

Poison ivy is everywhere . . . all over the United States, in fields and forests and your own backyard. You will know it by its shiny pointed leaves that grow in clusters of three. Sometimes it is a bit hard to recognize because it can grow as a plant, bush or vine.

Poison oak is less common. It looks much like poison ivy except that it has hairy leaves that resemble oak leaves.

You won't run into poison sumac unless you are in the swamps of the eastern U.S.

Look for a bush or a tree with two rows of small pointed leaves opposite each other and a leaflet at the tip.

All three of these poisonous plants have clusters of white shiny berries in the fall.

You can control the poison ivy in your yard by spraying it with herbicide every three weeks. But don't try to burn the plants, because the smoke and fumes can also cause an allergic reaction.

When you come into contact with any of these plants, first take off your clothes and wash the oil off your skin with soap and water as soon as you can.

Sponging with rubbing alcohol will help remove any remaining oil. Your clothes will need to be washed, too.

You can buy lotions and creams that will soothe the itch and help dry the rash without a prescription at your drugstore.

However, if your skin gets severely irritated or you find the rash on your face, you should see your doctor for treatment.

Delayed allergic reaction to insect stings

You think you're starting to have an allergic reaction but don't understand why.

Hives are breaking out and you feel flushed and itchy.

If a bee had just stung you, you would recognize the sting as the cause of this reaction.

But it has been two weeks since you encountered that wasp, and his sting didn't cause much of a problem then.

Could it possibly be significant now?

Yes, it certainly could.

Most reactions to insect stings are immediate — within minutes.

However, a recent study reported in *Emergency Medicine* (22,7:99) found that some individuals may experience an allergic reaction to a sting several hours or even days later.

Some New York doctors found that a group of their patients suffered typical allergic reactions up to fourteen days after being stung by insects.

Reactions varied but included some of the following symptoms: localized swelling at the site of the sting, itching, generalized skin rash, difficulty in breathing and painful swollen joints.

Patients who had been stung several times at once were a large part of the group with delayed reactions.

Therefore, many researchers think that a larger amount of insect venom might be a factor in a delayed reaction.

Some patients had allergic reactions at the time they were

stung and also experienced a second reaction several days later.

A very severe allergic reaction is called anaphylaxis. This means an over-reaction of a protective function.

Symptoms of anaphylaxis include rash, itching, swelling in the throat to the extent that the airway is obstructed, and circulatory difficulties.

If you think you're experiencing an allergic reaction that could be the result of an insect sting within the past couple of weeks, report this to your doctor immediately.

Your doctor might need to test you for hypersensitivity to insect venom.

If you are hypersensitive (or allergic) to insect stings, you will need to take proper precautions to avoid future stings and reactions.

Mild reactions serve as a warning that the next insect sting could be more serious, possibly even deadly.

Vitamin D cream for psoriasis

People with the dry, scaly skin disease known as psoriasis may find relief by using a skin cream containing an active form of vitamin D, according to a digest in *American Family Physician* (40,4:301).

More than three out of four psoriasis sufferers got consistent relief by applying calcitriol in a petroleum jelly base to the scaly areas.

Most got better without any side effects from the vitamin. Calcitrol is known medically as vitamin D3.

Liver trouble triggers skin disease

People with a history of liver disease run about a 60 percent higher risk of coming down with an unsightly skin disease, reports the *British Medical Journal* (300,6719:227).

The disease, lichen planus, causes thickened, scaly skin patches, often accompanied by persistent itching, on the arms, legs, stomach, chest, back and genital areas.

Gardeners' alert

If you have the South American lily *Alstroemeria* in your garden, always wear gloves when cutting stems and handling leaves, recommends *Science News* (137:11,174).

Alstroemeria produces a substance, called tuliposide, that caused itchy, scaly hands in 15 of 57 floral workers participating in a Pennsylvania study.

Mask out wart virus

If you have warts removed the space-age way — with a carbon dioxide laser beam — ask your doctor to give you a mask while he wears one at the same time.

Some people have developed warts in unusual areas like the nostrils, apparently because of inhaling the smoky vapor given off as the laser beam burns off the wart tissue.

The vapor in a few cases might contain enough of the human papillomavirus to generate a new infection elsewhere, says the digest in *Modern Medicine* (57,10:23).

Simple remedies for common skin disorders among the elderly

It can be a source of many compliments, or it can be a source of great irritation and embarrassment. The scientific word for it is "integument." The common word is "skin."

Elderly people who don't suffer from skin problems are usually delighted when someone comments on how young or healthy their skin looks. However, those fortunate people are in the minority.

More than half of all elderly people suffer from at least one skin problem or irritation from time to time. But, they don't have to suffer indefinitely, because some of the most common skin problems can be managed and treated very easily.

Xerosis, or dry skin, is one of the most common complaints among the elderly, reports the October 1990 *Geriatrics* (45,10:57). Dry skin is often the result of aging — oil and sweat glands no longer function as well as they should, and so they fail to keep the skin as moist as before.

However, there are several other factors that could cause dry skin: low humidity (occasionally caused by indoor heating and cooling), harsh soaps, and harsh weather (too much sun or wind exposure).

Finding relief for dry skin can be as simple as following a few easy guidelines:

1. Bathe in tepid (lukewarm) water instead of very hot water.

2. Avoid using harsh soaps or heavily scented or perfumed soaps. They strip the skin of its important oils and moisture.

3. Gently towel dry. Do not rub the skin with the towel. Instead, pat gently to avoid further chapping the sensitive skin.

4. Follow the bath with a generous application of a heavy moisturizing lotion or cream. Apply the lotion while the skin is still moist. (Putting lotion on dry skin can actually aggravate the situation. And, failure to apply any lotion at all also can aggravate the condition.)

Contact dermatitis is another common complaint among the elderly. This is an allergic reaction to some form of irritant that has come in contact with the skin. Irritants can include anything from fabric softeners and detergents, to dog or cat fur, to grass or hay.

1. The best way to treat allergic reactions is to avoid the irritant: change detergents, stop petting your neighbor's dog and wear garments with long sleeves when working in the yard.

2. Once the irritant is removed, consider using a mild hydrocortisone cream (a readily available over-the-counter product found at most pharmacies). Ask your pharmacist to recommend a mild hydrocortisone cream that will suit your needs. The pharmacist can assist you in choosing a cream that is both effective and safe to use.

3. Then follow the steps for dry skin relief.

Lichen simples chronicus is also a common skin irritation of the elderly. This condition involves a thickening and hardening of the skin caused by persistent rubbing and irritation. The most frequent sites of this skin problem are the arms, lower legs and back of the neck.

1. The most effective treatment for lichen simples chronicus is a stronger form of a hydrocortisone cream.

2. People who suffer from this skin condition must understand the "itch-and-scratch" cycle. The more you scratch, the more you injure the skin. The skin starts to heal, but healing skin itches. So, you scratch, and injure the skin again. To stop the cycle, you must stop scratching. The cortisone cream also helps the itching.

Skin problems can be very aggravating, but following a few simple steps usually will help clear up the problems right away.

If your skin problems continue after trying these home remedies, talk with your doctor. He can determine the next best course of action to help restore your skin to its healthy state.

Check your skin for warning signs: stop nutrition problems before they get started

You can watch your skin for signs of nutritional deficiencies that even your doctor might not see, reports Dr. Kenneth Neldner, chairman of the Dermatology Department at Texas Tech University.

Here are signs to watch for: scaly skin, canker sores, wounds that heal slowly and cracks in the corners of the mouth.

Researchers are discovering that even minor nutrition problems show up in the skin, sometimes long before a doctor might see the underlying cause, reports an article in the Dec. 4, 1990 *The Atlanta Journal*.

Here are some common deficiencies and their skin signs:

Vitamin C shortage — bleeding gums, soreness in mouth and gums, or a rough, scaly rash around hair roots.

Vitamin B complex deficiency — cracks and canker sores in the corners of the mouth.

Psoriasis and eczema — these skin problems might not be caused by nutrient shortages, but sometimes they can be successfully treated by taking fish oil. Fish oil contains fatty acids, which help the body fight inflammation caused by the two skin conditions.

Skin cancers — deficiencies in zinc, copper, selenium and vitamins A and E increase the risks of developing various skin cancers, the report says.

Because five out of six medical schools don't even offer a formal course in nutrition for medical students, many doctors don't recognize early signs of nutrition problems, says Dr. Neldner.

Don't try to medicate yourself.

If you have some of the possible early warning signs, tell your doctor about this nutritional research and ask that she look at your condition more closely.

Sleeping Problems

Insomnia — the sleeper's nightmare

We've all probably had a night or two when we just couldn't fall asleep — a minor inconvenience for most of us. But for some people, sleepless nights are a way of life.

The inability to fall asleep, a condition called insomnia, can lead to serious medical problems. One person even died after nine months without sleep.

"After [age] 60, people have more trouble falling asleep, awaken more often, and, once awake, find it more difficult, if not impossible, to drop back to sleep," according to a report in *FDA Consumer* (23,8:13-15).

Sleep needs vary from person to person. Adults sleep an average of seven and a half hours a night and need less sleep as they age, the report says.

Insomnia has a variety of causes: anxiety, stress, jet lag or too much caffeine or alcohol. Some medications may cause insomnia as well.

Is your sleeplessness serious? Ask yourself these questions:

• Do you always have trouble falling asleep? Are you still

awake a half hour after going to bed?

• Do you wake up several times during the night and have trouble falling back to sleep?

• Do you wake up early, after sleeping only a few hours?

If you answered yes to those questions, you may have insomnia. But don't panic. *FDA Consumer* offers several tips to help yourself get a good night's sleep:

• Cut down on caffeine intake, especially at night.

• Don't nap during the day.

• Take a warm bath before bedtime.

• Stick to a "sleep schedule," and don't sleep in on weekends.

• Avoid heavy meals before bedtime.

• Be sure your bedroom is at a comfortable temperature.

• Don't exercise before bedtime. (But regular exercise during the day will help you relax at night.)

Many people drink a glass of wine before bedtime, thinking it will help them relax. It often has the opposite effect, the report says.

If self-help remedies fail, a sleep clinic may be just the thing for you. There are more than 1,000 sleep clinics in the U.S. alone. Each is manned by teams of experts whose sole purpose is to find out why you can't sleep.

Usually, you must stay overnight in the clinic so that the research team can measure your brain activity, breathing and movements.

For a list of accredited sleep centers, write to: American Sleep Disorder Association, 604 Second St., S.W., Rochester, Minn. 55902.

Falling asleep the natural way

Of course, the safest way to fall asleep is without the help of

drugs. The *Health Letter* offers these tips:
- Don't nap during the day.
- Make your bedroom a quiet, restful place.
- Don't drink caffeinated beverages before bedtime.
- Try a warm bath, reading or eating a light snack just before bedtime. Go to bed the same time every night.

If you just cannot fall asleep without medication, use these precautions:
- Ask your doctor about specific side effects. If your doctor is not familiar with your history, tell him about all other medications you are currently taking. Some drugs can cause insomnia.
- Take the lowest dosage of sleeping medication possible.
- Don't have the prescription refilled.
- Don't drive, operate machinery or drink alcohol while taking sleeping medication.

Are doctors mistreating sleep problems, missing major illnesses?

It's a myth that aging itself causes insomnia and other sleep problems, say members of an expert government panel.

In fact, many doctors may be over-prescribing sleeping pills while missing more serious, underlying health problems in people over 65, says the report in *Medical World News* (31,8:38).

Poor sleep patterns might even be linked to increased fatalities, the report suggests.

A more helpful rule of thumb might be this, suggests Dr. Robert J. Joynt of the University of Rochester and chairman of the panel:

If you are over 65 and have trouble sleeping, something else probably is wrong with you — something other than just "getting old."

"Both prescription and nonprescription drugs may actually worsen sleep problems, as they deal with symptoms rather than underlying causes," the report says.

Two exceptions: pills work okay for sleeplessness caused by some psychiatric problems, stress and anxiety, and existing treatment helps sleep apnea, a form of breathing problem.

Usually, both the general public and doctors "have a poor understanding of sleep and its disorders," the National Institutes of Health panel says.

"The goal of therapy [for insomnia] should be to identify the underlying cause," the panel says.

Skimping on sleep can shorten your life span

Could you be taking eight to ten years off your life span by not getting enough sleep at night? Experts are beginning to think so.

Nearly 50 percent of all Americans (five out of every 10 people) short themselves one to two hours of sleep each night. Each night adds up, and by the end of the week, it's as if you missed a whole night of sleep!

The typical 24-hour on-the-go schedule that most Americans keep these days is resulting in a nation of "walking zombies", says a recent report in *The Atlanta Journal* (108,22).

Researchers now are recognizing the consequences of sleepiness: loss of initiative, loss of energy, attention lapses, distractibility and fatigue.

Researchers also report that after five years, people who work night shifts and don't get enough sleep are twice as likely to suffer from heart ailments and gastrointestinal diseases than those who work day shifts and get enough sleep.

"There's even evidence that people getting inadequate sleep shorten their life span by eight to 10 years," reports Dr. James Maas, a researcher from Cornell University.

Here's a simple test to see if you need more sleep: if you need an alarm clock to get up in the morning, or if you feel more than just a minor sag in the middle of the day, you probably need more sleep.

Snorer alert — you may be suffering from sleep apnea

If you snore, are tired in the morning and sleepy throughout the day, you might be suffering from sleep apnea (pronounced **ap**-nee-a).

Apnea is a medical problem that causes people to stop breathing at least five times during the night for periods of 20 to 40 seconds each time.

These stoppages decrease the supply of oxygen to the brain, resulting in sleepiness and loss of concentration during waking hours, especially in the evening.

Typical sufferers are middle-aged and elderly men who are loud snorers and overweight, says a report from the American Lung Association.

The most common cause of sleep apnea is obesity.

Being too fat causes an excessive amount of soft tissue to accumulate in the throat, resulting in an obstructed airway, snoring and apnea.

If you lose weight and quit smoking, you probably will eliminate the underlying cause of apnea, says a report in *British Medical Journal* (298,6678:904).

The most annoying symptom of sleep apnea — for people who live with you, that is — is snoring.

Here are a few tips for snorers from sleep experts:

• Prop your head up at night before falling asleep.

• If you snore only while lying on your back, a tennis ball sewn into the back of your pajama top will prompt you to roll over onto your side or stomach.

• If you think your problem is beyond your control, see your doctor, who can bring you up-to-date on the latest medical techniques to treat sleeping disorders.

Surgery to correct apnea is a last resort.

Sleep apnea may be underlying cause of some dementia

Some elderly people have a sleep disorder called sleep apnea. Many of them don't know they have this enemy of a good night's rest.

Now, researchers are finding that sleep apnea might be the villain behind some cases of mental deterioration that seem like senility, says a report in *Geriatrics* (45,6:16).

The higher the number of episodes of sleep apnea, the poorer some elderly people performed on tests of mental and physical abilities, according to Dr. D.L. Bliwise of the Sleep Disorders Center at Stanford Medical School in California.

These are the same tests given to people to find out if they have Alzheimer's disease or other forms of mental deterioration.

The researcher believes that sleep apnea might be the underlying cause of some cases of mental declines.

Treating the apnea might reverse the mental deterioration in some people, Bliwise hopes.

It's not a case of sleeping longer, but of sleeping better.

People with sleep apnea tend to snore a lot, and loudly.

More dangerously, they actually stop breathing for periods ranging from a few seconds to more than a minute at a time.

It's almost as if they "forget" to breathe. Soft tissue in the breathing passage relaxes and acts like a trapdoor, shutting off the air. That can happen many times a night.

Sometimes they wake up suddenly with a sensation of having lost their breath or of choking without air.

Such episodes result in a lighter, "restless" sleep.

It's not hard to see how a breathless, restless night could mess up your next day, and even dull your thinking after a while.

If you snore a lot, you might have sleep apnea.

Check with your doctor about the treatments available for this potentially serious disorder.

Getting the most out of your rest

Your doctor tells you to get more rest. So you go to bed a little earlier. But you lie awake until the wee hours of the morning. And after you finally fall asleep, you wake up feeling just as tired as you did when you went to bed. Sound familiar?

You and millions of other elderly men and women are not getting as much out of their rest time as they should.

However, following a few simple suggestions will help make sure your rest time is truly restful.

1. Play soft, relaxing music while you rest or before you go to bed to help you unwind from the day.

2. Take bedtime medications one or two hours before you go to bed, if your doctor has prescribed them for you.

3. Take pain relievers and other medications on the schedule that your doctor recommends. Sticking to the schedule helps keep a steady, effective amount of medicine in your body at all times, so you'll be less likely to be awakened by pain or discomfort.

4. Sleep on a firm mattress for good back support.

5. Try to avoid caffeine, especially close to bedtime. It interferes with sleep.

6. Avoid alcohol. It may make you sleepy at bedtime, but it often leaves you wide awake at 2 or 3 a.m. It can also interfere with medications.

7. Go to sleep and rise on a regular schedule. And try to sleep at least five to six hours each night.

8. Exercise enough each day to stay flexible and to keep good muscle tone. It is very easy to "stiffen up" if you don't do some exercise. You and your doctor can plan an effective and fun exercise program to suit your needs.

9. Take warm baths or use gentle massage to relieve joint or muscle aches and pains.

Following these simple suggestions on a regular, long-term basis will help you get the most out of your rest time.

And getting the most out of your rest time will help you make the most out of your day.　　　Source: *Senior Patient* (2,1:57).

Fool your body: day and night can become just like night and day

If your eyelids are at half-mast only two hours into your night shift, but you're having trouble sleeping when you finally get home in the morning, you may need to "fool" your body clock.

Harvard researchers have found a way for night shift workers to do just that.

According to a report in *The New England Journal of Medicine* (322, 18:1253), you should work under extremely bright lights (comparable to sunlight) during the night shift. This fools your body into thinking it's daytime.

Then you need to cover your windows with dark curtains to sleep during the day, so that you fool your body into thinking it's night.

By the fourth or fifth day of this routine, your internal body clock will have shifted.

Resetting your internal body clock should help you stay alert during the night while you're at work and help you sleep better during the day.

Strokes

Daily aspirin dose could reduce your risk of stroke

If you suffer from abnormal fluttering of the heart, you have a high risk of stroke; and a daily dose of aspirin might dramatically reduce your risk, according to a special report in *The New England Journal of Medicine* (322,12:863).

Researchers studied 1,244 men and women with atrial fibrillation, the medical term for heart flutter. They discovered that aspirin cut the risk of stroke by 50 to 80 percent, the report stated.

Those findings also held true for an anti-clotting drug, warfarin, which is available only by prescription.

Researchers estimate that of the one million elderly people with atrial fibrillation, 75,000 will suffer a stroke this year.

In the on-going studies, begun in 1987, heart-patient volunteers have been taking aspirin, warfarin or a placebo (a harmless substance that only looks like a real drug).

Among the people taking warfarin or aspirin, only 1.6 percent have suffered strokes, compared with 8.3 percent of the people taking the placebo, the study reports.

Those dramatic results have prompted researchers to switch placebo patients to aspirin or warfarin.

Researchers found that people taking 325-milligram tablets of aspirin daily have cut their stroke risk by nearly 50 percent compared with placebo patients.

Many strokes happen when a blood clot blocks a blood vessel in the brain. Researchers believe aspirin and warfarin prevent strokes by making blood less "sticky," reducing its tendency to clot.

Aspirin and warfarin seem to work better at preventing minor, "minimally disabling" strokes than at stopping fatal ones.

Although the preliminary findings seem encouraging, so far the study has failed to show that aspirin benefits people over age 75.

Researchers don't know why, although previous studies have suggested that people over age 75 may have more diseases that increase their risk of stroke.

And the alternative treatment, warfarin, generally is not recommended for those elderly patients, researchers say.

"The results must be interpreted cautiously ... in view of the limited duration of follow-up, which to date averages little more than one year per patient," researchers say in the report.

They plan to follow up study patients every three months to determine the difference in benefits between aspirin and warfarin.

They will also look at long-term effects of both drugs.

Previous studies have shown aspirin's ability to ward off heart attacks and migraine pain when taken every day.

Before you start taking an aspirin a day, check with your doctor.

Don't medicate yourself without getting good medical advice first.

Stroke recovery hampered by some medications

Certain medications, if given shortly after a stroke, can slow down a patient's recovery, according to a report in *Medical World News* (31,6:11).

Dr. Larry B. Goldstein and his colleagues at Duke University Medical Center, Durham, N.C., studied the records of 58 stroke patients to determine the effects of different drugs on recovery.

Of the 58 patients, 24 took *clonidine* (a drug used to lower high blood pressure) at the time of their stroke or during their treatment. Patients who did not take clonidine improved more quickly than those who did.

Dr. Goldstein said he does not give stroke patients *haloperidol* (an antipsychotic drug) or *diazepam* (a tranquilizer), stating, "We're just starting to learn which drugs can be harmful under what circumstances."

Corn oil is latest weapon in war against strokes

Olive oil may be great in your Greek salad, but corn oil might be better for your heart.

Corn oil seems to be able to lower the level of plasma fibrinogen in the blood, reports the August 1990 *Journal of the American College of Nutrition* (9,4:352).

Plasma fibrinogen is a kind of protein in the blood that helps make blood "sticky" and form clots. Too much fibrinogen causes the blood to "thicken" and clot abnormally.

Abnormal clotting is unhealthy and may contribute to strokes, atherosclerosis (hardening of the arteries) and heart disease.

Since some oils seem to lower the amount of fibrinogen, scientists wanted to find out which one does the best job: dietary fish oil, corn oil or olive oil.

They fed the oils to three groups of volunteers for eight weeks and then tallied the results.

The fish oil group and the corn oil group were number one and two in lowering plasma fibrinogen. Olive oil was least effective and came in third.

Researchers already knew that fish oil lowers fibrinogen levels. But, what's new is the discovery that corn oil also does a good job in making blood more "slippery" and less liable to stick together in clots.

Corn oil might become the latest nutritional weapon against strokes and heart disease, the report suggests.

Thyroid Problems

Thyroid activity: too much or too little can be dangerous

If you suffer from constipation, brittle nails and dry skin, ask your doctor to check your thyroid gland, advises Dr. David Cooper in *Medical World News* (30,19:54).

These three symptoms might be indications of an underactive thyroid gland, otherwise known as hypothyroidism.

Other markers include fatigue, depression and coarse hair.

People over 60 are twice as likely to have an underactive thyroid gland as younger people, according to the report.

This "sub-clinical" form of hypothyroidism affects about two of every 10 women and one of every 10 men past middle age.

The condition is commonly misdiagnosed in elderly people, Dr. Cooper adds.

The thyroid gland is about the size of a walnut and is located at the base of the neck near the windpipe.

It produces hormones that, when released into the bloodstream, help the body convert oxygen and nutrients into energy.

An underactive thyroid gland doesn't produce enough hormones to keep your energy levels high.

On the other hand, an overactive thyroid gland produces too many hormones, resulting in nervousness and diarrhea.

That condition is known as hyperthyroidism.

Think of it this way — "hypo" is too little and "hyper" is too much.

One reason for misdiagnosis, Dr. Cooper says, is disagreement on the normal hormone levels for elderly people.

As you age, your thyroid gland naturally may produce more hormones.

However, this increased production of hormones still may not meet your body's needs, the report indicates.

But the increased production may fool your doctor, who may say that your thyroid is functioning normally.

Hypothyroidism is easily treated with hormone-replacement therapy, Dr. Cooper says.

Two cautions: this therapy may cause mineral loss from bones. For those with osteoporosis, the "brittle-bone" disease, such therapy could make a bad condition worse.

And second, taking extra thyroid hormone could tip you over into hyperthyroidism — too much thyroid hormone.

The treatment must be closely monitored by your doctor.

Symptoms of hypothyroidism resemble menopause

Feeling unusually tired and fatigued? Suffering from dry skin and thinning hair? Tired of that puffiness around the eyes?

Yes, you say, I am tired of all those things, but my doctor told me to expect these things during menopause.

Well, menopause might not be the problem.

You could be suffering from hypothyroidism — a condition

in which the thyroid gland produces an abnormally small amount of its hormones.

Hypothyroidism is often misdiagnosed or underdiagnosed, especially among menopausal women, because its symptoms resemble other common disorders, warns a recent report in the *Medical Tribune* (31, 21: 2).

Menopausal women often mistake the symptoms of hypothyroidism for the symptoms of menopause. These symptoms include fatigue, impaired memory, dry skin, thinning hair, puffy eyes and depression.

Even if the doctor suspects and tests for hypothyroidism, the true results of the thyroxine tests are often "hidden" by estrogen therapy. Apparently, estrogen therapy can cause an abnormal thyroid test to look normal.

Researchers suggest that doctors should test for levels of thyroid stimulating hormone (TSH). This hormone level can accurately tell if the thyroid is functioning properly without the result being masked by estrogen therapy.

Urinary Problems

Don't be embarrassed to discuss UTI with your doctor

Discussing a urinary tract infection (UTI) with your doctor may be embarrassing, but it's necessary. If left untreated, a UTI could damage your kidneys, according to *Lifetime Health Letter* (2,3:3).

UTIs affect nearly five million Americans a year and occur in both men and women, although they are more common in women after menopause.

UTIs are caused by bacteria, and one reason women are reluctant to talk to their doctor is that the infection is often sexually related. (Some women feel discomfort when urinating as early as one day after sexual intercourse.)

The bacteria that cause the infection lie dormant in the body and somehow make their way to the urinary tract, causing infection.

The type of contraceptive used can also increase UTI risk.

"Women who use diaphragms have considerably more UTIs than women who use oral contraceptives," according to the report. Contraceptive foams and condoms also increase the risk slightly.

A UTI can come on quickly and without warning. Its symptoms include the need to urinate more often, and a burning sensation during urination.

UTIs can be treated effectively with antibiotics, but you must see your doctor right away, especially if you've had UTIs before. Often, your doctor can do a simple test in the office rather than sending a urine sample to a laboratory. Many women who are prone to UTIs take small, regular amounts of antibiotics to ward off infections.

There are many myths regarding urinary tract infections. One is that drinking cranberry juice will cure a UTI. Not true. Although the acid in cranberry juice can kill bacteria, you'd have to drink several gallons of it.

But drinking lots of water after intercourse will help prevent UTIs.

"In effect, you're washing away the bacteria before they have a chance to cause an infection," according to the report. You should also urinate frequently throughout the day, rather than "hold it."

So far, studies have failed to show that bubble baths, hot tubs and swimming pools contribute to urinary tract infections.

Urinary tract infections bring misery and possible danger to kidneys

Embarrassing to talk about, impossible to live with, and painful enough to cause five million doctor visits yearly — the urinary tract infection is a nightmare for 20 percent of the female population, says a report in *The Annals of Internal Medicine* (111,11:906).

The entire urinary tract can become infected by invading bacteria, but the bladder is most often pin-pointed, especially in women. Unhappily, one infection seems to spawn others, so your first infection probably won't be your last.

Women are the primary target of recurring urinary tract infections due in large part to sexual intercourse. This makes some women feel awkward talking to their doctor about the frequency of their infections.

Pain and discomfort from UTIs can appear quickly. Some women report symptoms as early as the day following sexual activity.

Symptoms often vary, depending on the location of the infection, but two common complaints are a frequent need to urinate and pain during intercourse.

Most often the pain is described as a burning sensation, although some women complain of a "stomachache" right below the naval area, where the bladder is located.

Women past the age of menopause are especially prone to infections. This seems to be attributable to the thinning of vaginal and urethral tissues brought about by menopause.

Fortunately, most of these women respond to the addition of estrogen in the form of hormone-replacement therapy.

Since UTIs can mimic other medical problems, such as vaginal inflammation, it is important to see a doctor for an accurate diagnosis.

Most doctors have the necessary lab equipment to confirm an infection, thereby ensuring proper and prompt medical attention.

Since urinary infections generally respond quickly to antibiotics, the key is to seek professional help as soon as symptoms first appear.

Doctors sometimes prescribe small amounts of medication to be taken as a preventative measure to women who have seemingly "constant" infections.

When left untreated, the urinary tract infection can spread to the kidneys, where the potential for kidney damage can then turn the UTI into a serious health problem.

Many doctors suggest drinking several glasses of water each day to help prevent UTIs. Drinking a lot of water causes frequent urination, which helps "wash away" the bacteria before they have time to cause an infection.

Urinary incontinence in the elderly

It's troublesome, aggravating, and, most of all, embarrassing. And it affects at least 10 million adults in the United States today — urinary incontinence.

It is defined as "the involuntary loss of urine so severe as to have social and/or hygienic consequences." It is a problem that should not be taken lightly or ignored.

The complications of urinary incontinence include rashes, sores and skin and urinary tract infections. People who suffer from urinary incontinence also experience limitations in social activities, which can lead to isolation and depression.

According to a report in *U.S. Pharmacist* (15,3:58), there are several different kinds of urinary incontinence.

1. **Stress incontinence** is the leakage of small amounts of urine that occurs when laughing, coughing, or sneezing.

2. **Urge incontinence** is the most common form of incontinence in the elderly. Those who suffer from this type experience a sudden need to urinate, but cannot hold the urine long enough to reach a toilet. Usually only a small amount of

urine is lost, but this may occur every few hours.

3. **Overflow incontinence** consists of a fairly continuous flow of urine — also known as "dribbling."

4. **Functional incontinence** involves losing a large amount of urine all at once. The problem here lies in physical or mental handicaps — the person either cannot physically get to the bathroom in time, or he doesn't mentally recognize the need to urinate until it is too late.

5. **Mixed incontinence** usually involves a combination of stress and urge incontinence. This form is common in the elderly.

Although some cases of incontinence must be treated with drugs or surgery, there are some simple at-home remedies that may help in the management of incontinence.

1. **Pelvic muscle exercises** (Kegel exercises) strengthen the muscles that help control urine flow. To perform these exercises, contract the muscles that will stop the flow of urine. Do this ten times, relax, then do ten more. Gradually increase the number you do each day. Do this several times a day for several minutes at a time. Do not do many of these on the first day — you'll be sore the next day. Kegel exercises are successful in helping with incontinence in 30 - 90 percent of all women.

2. **Biofeedback** is useful for management of stress and urge incontinence. People are trained to have better control over the storage of urine (check with your doctor for more information on this training).

3. **Bladder training** helps people control incontinence by training them to void at regular intervals. Gradually, the intervals are lengthened to a maximum point that each individual can maintain. This remedy is especially helpful in urge and stress incontinence, and most people experience some relief using this method.

4. **Palliative treatment** doesn't actually "treat" the incontinence, but it helps people feel less socially isolated. This treatment involves the use of absorbent products (Depends, Serenity), external collecting devices for men (Texas or condom catheters) and bed pads.

These simple remedies may be helpful in the management of urinary incontinence. However, they are not a substitute for a medical evaluation.

If you have any trouble with urinary incontinence, check with your doctor immediately to determine the cause and discuss possible treatments.

Urinary incontinence is a nuisance, but it doesn't have to be a permanent handicap.

The combination of your doctor's advice and simple at-home remedies can help you manage the problem and resume your normal daily activities.

Vascular and Circulatory Problems

Risk factors for phlebitis and blood clots

If you sit much of the time, or spend hours on your feet without other exercise, you may be at high risk for phlebitis.

That's a painful condition in which a vein becomes inflamed, and a blood clot forms.

Clots, especially in the large leg veins, are dangerous. Sometimes clots break up and travel to the lungs or heart, causing serious damage or death.

Phlebitis most often affects the legs, although it can occur anywhere in the body, says Dr. Thomas Riles, a surgeon at New York University Medical Center.

Leg injuries sometimes trigger phlebitis, but clots usually develop when people don't get enough exercise to keep blood circulating in their legs.

Police officers, teachers, and bedridden patients are commonly affected.

Phlebitis is more common in older people, and women get it

more often than men.

Phlebitis can occur in veins close to the skin — superficial veins—or in veins deeper in the body. The deeper ones cause the most trouble.

Blood clots in superficial veins look like knots or cords and are easily seen. The vein is painful and tender.

Deep-vein phlebitis causes severe pain and may involve the entire leg, not just the vein. The calf or thigh may swell and turn blue.

The good news is that phlebitis is preventable. Here are some tips from Dr. Riles:

- If you stand for long hours while on the job or have varicose veins, wear support hosiery.

- While traveling, be sure to stretch every half hour. A short walk will help keep blood circulating in your legs.

- Consider losing weight. Overweight people are more likely to suffer from phlebitis.

You can ease the pain by elevating your legs and taking aspirin. Warm compresses will also help.

If infection sets in, your doctor will prescribe antibiotics.

In all cases of suspected phlebitis, see your doctor immediately. This can be a very serious condition.

Exercise decreases risk of blood clots

A walk in the park may be just what your body needs to help protect you from dangerous blood clots. According to a recent report in *The Physician and Sportsmedicine* (18,3:43), regular exercise increases your body's ability to dissolve blood clots.

A study at the University of Washington in Seattle shows that exercising regularly increases the activity of TPA (tissue plasminogen activator) in the body.

TPA is a protein substance in the body that dissolves blood clots and reduces your chances of developing blood clots.

Dr. John Stratton from the University of Washington studied 16 healthy men from ages 25-74 for six months.

The subjects were placed on walking, jogging or bicycling programs for the six months to observe the effects of regular exercise.

At the end of the six months, the researchers measured the amount of TPA in the blood, and they found a significant increase of TPA in the blood, especially in the older men.

In fact, some of the older men experienced as much as a 39 percent increase in the amount of TPA in their blood. The greater amount of TPA in the blood reduces the risk of forming blood clots.

Dr. Stratton's study also showed that fibrin, a protein which causes blood clots, decreased by about 14 percent with regular exercise.

Since the protein fibrin actually promotes blood clots, the researchers noted that fibrin is "a clear-cut risk factor (for blood clots) in the same order of magnitude as cholesterol."

And scientists say that high levels of fibrin have been connected to deaths from heart disease.

Since regular exercise reduced the amount of fibrin in the blood, the exercisers obviously had a decreased chance of developing blood clots.

The combined effects of more TPA and less fibrin in the blood work together to help protect people from blood clots and heart disease or strokes.

Therefore, people who formulate an exercise program with their doctor have a great chance of preventing blood clots and avoiding heart attacks and strokes.

Researchers also have found that regular exercise can help regulate the levels of TPA and fibrin in the blood after a heart attack and help reduce the risk of a second heart attack.

Doctors say that other benefits of a regular exercise program, in addition to the reduced risk of heart disease, are lowered blood pressure, a decrease in body fat and an increase in beneficial HDL (high density lipoprotein) cholesterol levels.

Check with your doctor to develop an exercise program that is best for you.

Polycythemia vera

The deep red skin color in Uncle Jake that you always attributed to good health and extra sunshine possibly could be the hallmark sign of a serious blood disorder known as polycythemia vera.

This blood disorder causes the body to produce too many red blood cells, and the disorder could be life-threatening if not recognized and treated immediately.

Here's the catch — polycythemia is treatable, but it is very hard to recognize and diagnose.

The most obvious symptoms of the disease are often confused with other less-dangerous conditions.

The most obvious symptom is a gradual change in skin color from the normal flesh color to various shades of red.

According to *The Journal of the American Medical Association* (263,18:2481), the change in skin color is so gradual that it is often overlooked. The high red color is usually thought to be from robust health or exposure to the elements.

Bloodshot eyes are another symptom of polycythemia vera. However, people often mistake them for conjunctivitis, allergies or overindulgence in alcohol.

A symptom that is unique to this disorder is pruritus (severe itching), which is occasionally aggravated by bathing. Other symptoms may include mental sluggishness, lethargy, weakness and fatigue.

The dangers of polycythemia vera, if left untreated, are the risks of thrombosis (blood clots, which could lead to strokes and heart attacks), ulcers and intestinal hemorrhages. The longer the disorder is untreated, the greater the risk of these conditions.

The good news is that polycythemia vera can be treated and managed effectively to insure a normal life-style.

Check with your doctor for answers to questions about the diagnosis and treatment of polycythemia vera.

Relief from Raynaud's

Raynaud's disease is associated with a decreased blood flow to the fingers and toes.

The fingers or toes turn blue or white, with some degree of numbness, and they rewarm very slowly.

Raynaud's sufferers have always been advised to wear warm socks and gloves in the wintertime, but now scientists have devised a new at-home treatment plan to help manage the symptoms, says a recent report in *The Physician and Sports-medicine* (18,3:129).

The steps for this procedure are as follows:

1. Fill two bowls with water of about 120 degrees. Place one bowl in a cold area (either a room or outdoors), and place the other in a warm room.

2. Dress lightly, as you would for room temperature. In the warm room, put both hands in the 120-degree water for two to five minutes.

3. Wrap the hands in a towel and go to the cold room. Again put both hands in the 120-degree water for two to five minutes.

4. Repeat step 2 — put hands in warm water in the warm room for two to five minutes.

5. Repeat this procedure three to six times a day for a total of about 50 trials.

Following these simple steps can give relief from the problems of Raynaud's disease.

Salt causes brain damage?

Too much salt in your diet may be harmful to more than just your blood pressure.

According to *Science News* (137,15:238), researchers think that salt may cause brain tissue damage.

Apparently, too much salt in the diet damages and narrows artery walls.

These narrow arteries cut off blood supplies to the brain, which results in brain tissue damage and could lead to a stroke.

Maintaining a low-salt diet can decrease the risk of brain tissue damage.

CHAPTER TWENTY-FIVE

Vitamin E helps reverse damage from hardening of the arteries

If you're suffering from atherosclerosis, or you have a family history of atherosclerosis (hardening of the arteries) and you fear that you might develop it, vitamin E might be the vitamin for you.

Vitamin E is taking a leading role in the fight against atherosclerosis, reports a recent digest in the October 1990 *Nutrition Today* (25,5:5).

Based on recent studies, vitamin E seems to help prevent the development of atherosclerosis, and it also seems to help reduce the damage if atherosclerosis has already begun.

The study reports that lab animals that were fed diets without vitamin E had about 79 percent more artery blockage than those animals fed the same diet but containing vitamin E.

Researchers also fed vitamin E enriched diets to lab animals that had been suffering from atherosclerosis for at least one year. After two years on a diet rich in vitamin E, the animals went from having 35 percent artery blockage to 15 percent.

Large amounts of vitamin E can be harmful, so never take vitamin E supplements without first talking to your doctor.

Vitamins and Minerals

Blood vessel disease — "B"-ware!

If your doctor has warned you about your risk of strokes or blood vessel diseases, but you're not suffering from high cholesterol levels, vitamin B may be just what you need.

The American Heart Association reports that a metabolic defect that can lead to blood vessel disease and increase the risk of stroke may be corrected with vitamin B supplements.

The defect is known as "mild hyperhomocysteinemia." This condition results in slight to moderate elevations of homocysteine, an amino acid that circulates in the blood.

At normal levels, this amino acid is harmless. But research indicates that mildly elevated levels may damage blood vessels and possibly lead to atherosclerosis or "hardening of the arteries."

The American Heart Association reports that excess homocysteine seems to damage blood vessels. Homocysteine causes sores and scars to form on blood vessel walls, similar to how cholesterol does.

If a blood clot forms on the lesions and blocks blood flow to the heart or brain, it can trigger a heart attack or stroke.

The good news is that vitamin B can help break down extra homocysteine in the blood and prevent dangerous build-ups of the amino acid.

B vitamins (biotin, B6, B12) convert the homocysteine to a harmless kind of amino acid called methionine.

Eliminating the extra homocysteine from the blood greatly reduces risk of blood vessel diseases.

People who have suffered from hardening of the arteries that could not be explained by high cholesterol levels are the most likely suspects for mild hyperhomocysteinemia.

But don't try to treat yourself without your doctor's advice!

If you're concerned about your risk of blood vessel disease, talk to your doctor about the best type of therapy for you.

Megadoses of slow-release niacin could damage your liver

Slow-release forms of niacin in large doses could damage your liver, warn two recent reports in *The Journal of the American Medical Association* (264,2:181 and 241).

Doctors have known for a long time that megadoses of niacin, also known as vitamin B3, can cause liver failure.

But until now, some had believed that people needing large doses of niacin might be better off taking the sustained-release tablets, the kind that dissolve slowly in the body and feed out smaller levels of the vitamin over many hours.

According to the July 11 report in *JAMA*, four people developed serious liver damage after taking the slow-release niacin instead of the crystalline form.

Two of them changed from the prescribed crystalline kind to the slow-release kind — one 62-year-old man on his own initiative and a 47-year-old man on a pharmacists's recommendation.

In a third case, a doctor prescribed slow-release niacin for a 50-year-old woman.

All three had been receiving doctor-prescribed treatment of high-dose niacin to lower their high cholesterol levels. They had been taking between 1,500 milligrams and 4,000 milligrams of niacin daily under doctors' supervision.

The fourth said he had been taking one 500-milligram slow-release niacin tablet daily for two months as a supplement without checking with a doctor.

The Recommended Dietary Allowance for niacin is 15 milligrams per day for men over 50, and 13 milligrams daily for women over 50.

Normally, doctors prescribe the crystalline form of niacin, known as nicotinic acid (no relation whatsoever to the drug nicotine found in tobacco).

Niacin in high doses — sometimes 100 or more times the RDA — is very effective in lowering excessive levels of cholesterol in the blood.

The problem is that such high-dose niacin can cause unpleasant side effects, such as skin flushing, especially of the face, and widespread itching.

In addition, a person taking such high doses can suffer liver damage, even while under the close supervision of a doctor.

The slow-release form cuts down on the flushing and itching. But it apparently is more dangerous to the liver, in lower doses and over shorter periods of time.

Slow-release niacin tablets are available without prescription in many health food stores and pharmacies.

Such cases point out again the wisdom of checking first with your doctor before taking supplements of any kind.

Be especially cautious about taking megadoses of vitamins and minerals that are far beyond recommended daily needs.

Some megadoses can be dangerous, even deadly.

More niacin cautions

■ High-dose niacin, in whatever form it's taken, is a drug, not a vitamin anymore, warns Denise Arthurs of the Tufts University Nutrition Center in Boston.

"At the levels recommended by popular [nutrition] books and by people in the lay public — 1,500, 2,000, 3,000 milligrams — niacin ceases to be a vitamin and is, in fact, a drug," Arthurs says. "It has side effects like most drugs do."

She urged that such high doses be taken only under the direction and constant monitoring of a doctor, reports *Medical Tribune* (31,16:14).

■ Niacin in high doses should be avoided by some diabetics, warns a recent report in *The Journal of the American Medical Association* (264,6:723).

Megadose niacin dramatically lowers cholesterol levels, including LDL ("bad") cholesterol.

But, people with non-insulin-dependent diabetes may suffer from a niacin side-effect, the report says.

Niacin treatment in this form of diabetes causes a loss of control of blood sugar levels.

The researchers recommended caution in using nicotinic acid for these diabetics.

Low selenium levels linked to cancers, asthma, digestive ills

■ Men seem to be more sensitive to a deficiency of the mineral nutrient selenium.

Men with lower levels of selenium in their blood were more likely to develop cancers of the lung, stomach and pancreas, reports the *Journal of the National Cancer Institute* (82,10:864).

That finding comes from a big, 10-year Finnish study of nearly 40,000 men and women.

Women had a marginally higher risk because of low selenium, but not nearly so much as men, according to researcher Paul Knekt.

Men who averaged 59.1 micrograms of selenium per liter of blood had the highest risk. Men with an average of 62.5 micrograms had the lowest risk, the report says.

People in Finland, a Scandinavian country bordering the Soviet Union, don't get much selenium in their diets, the report says.

The U.S. Recommended Dietary Allowance (RDA) for selenium is 70 micrograms daily for men over 50, and 55 micrograms for women 51 and above.

■ Low selenium levels also seem to be linked in some way to bladder cancer.

Thirty-five people developed bladder cancer out of a group of 25,802 people that researchers were keeping tabs on.

Those with bladder cancer had significantly lower blood levels of selenium than people who were cancer-free, according to a digest of a study in *Cancer Research* (49,21:6144).

■ In another Scandinavian country, Sweden, researchers measured blood levels of selenium in people who were being treated for diseases of the heart and digestive system.

The biggest shortages were found among those with digestive diseases.

People with stomach and intestinal diseases might have selenium deficiency, the report indicates. A selenium shortage could further harm their immune systems and delay their recovery.

They might need selenium supplements, the report suggests.

■ Two studies suggest that low selenium levels might contribute to the development of asthma or even partly cause it.

People with symptoms of asthma have lower levels of selenium in their blood and blood plasma, says a British study reported in *Clinical Science* (77,5:495).

In New Zealand, people with the lowest levels of selenium are twice as likely to develop asthma as those with the highest levels.

Also, those with low levels of glutathione peroxidase had five times the asthma risk, says a study in the British scientific journal *Thorax* (45:95).

Glutathione peroxidase is a natural anti-inflammatory enzyme produced by the body.

Selenium forms part of the chemical makeup of this enzyme, which battles the inflammation of lung tissues caused by asthma.

A New Zealander typically gets less than 30 micrograms a day of selenium.

■ Selenium apparently works closely with vitamin E, a powerful antioxidant, to neutralize harmful free radicals circulating in the blood.

Natural sources of selenium include Brazil nuts, salmon, tuna, swordfish, shrimp, lobster, oysters, whole grains and sunflower seeds.

Brazil nuts are an especially rich source, mainly because they are grown in soil high in selenium.

In fact, a quarter-ounce of Brazil nut meat — about the size of one nut — provides 76.8 micrograms of selenium, well above the RDA.

But, be aware that one Brazil nut is about 85 percent fat, one-third of that saturated fat.

Check with your doctor before taking a selenium supplement.

Even small amounts above the RDA can cause side effects like nail damage, hair loss, nausea, diarrhea, skin odor, fatigue, irritability and even damage to the nervous system, says *Recommended Dietary Allowances, 10th Edition* (National Research Council, 1989:pg.221).

Pills' crumbling and dissolving times are important

Have your calcium supplements passed the vinegar test?

If not, your body might not be getting the benefit of what you're feeding it, suggests a report in *Nutrition Action Health Letter* (17,5:1).

The vinegar test can show how quickly and completely your calcium tablet crumbles and dissolves.

If your tablet flunks the test in vinegar, it probably won't dissolve in your body either, says the report.

Here's how to find out whether you're getting the nutrients you're paying for:

Put one tablet in a glass of plain apple-cider vinegar. That's to simulate the acid environment of your stomach, the first stop for anything you take by mouth.

Time how long it takes the tablet to completely disintegrate (crumble apart).

In addition, measure how long it takes for the crumbled tablet to dissolve in the liquid and become part of the liquid solution.

Crumbling time of an hour or more might indicate a problem.

If the tablet hasn't crumbled by the time it leaves your stomach, the calcium carbonate probably won't get absorbed into your bloodstream, says the *Nutrition Action* report.

Dissolving time of more than a half-day should be a warning sign, whether regular or timed-release forms of calcium.

Try a similar test with your other vitamin-mineral supplements.

Drop a tablet into just a glass of plain water.

Again, if it takes more than four or five hours to dissolve, much, if not most, of the nutrients will just pass on through your system without getting absorbed.

"Tablets that do disintegrate may not get into the bloodstream," the reports quotes University of Maryland researcher Ralph Shangraw. "But if it doesn't disintegrate, that's a pretty good indication that it won't get absorbed."

Shangraw calls for much quicker crumbling times — under 30 minutes.

Some brands do better than others.

Supplements with potentially poor dissolving rates include generic-brand multi-vitamins and multi-minerals, timed- or slow-release tablets and big, solid pills like calcium-magnesium-zinc combinations.

Some slow-release tablets may not dissolve at all.

The report tells of one supplement user who opened his septic tank for repair and discovered a layer of undissolved vitamin pills.

Generally, capsules out-perform solid tablets or pills, usually because capsules have a gelatin outer-skin that dissolves quickly in the stomach.

Liquid forms, of course, are the most quickly absorbed.

Severe form of leukemia halted with vitamin A drug

French researchers report promising results in treating a severe kind of blood cancer with a concentrated form of vitamin A.

Using retinoic acid, a derivative of vitamin A, three out of four people with acute myeloid leukemia were disease-free up to nine months after treatment stopped, according to a report in *The Lancet* (2,8665:746).

Vegetarians need vitamins

People on strict vegetarian diets may run a greater risk of developing vitamin B12 and vitamin D deficiencies than non-vegetarians.

According to a report in *The American Journal of Clinical Nutrition* (50,4:718), a recent French study indicates that vegetarians and non-vegetarians had equal amounts of thiamin, riboflavin, folates and vitamins B6, A, and E.

However, the vegetarians had lower amounts of vitamin B-12 and vitamin D than the non-vegetarians.

To prevent vitamin deficiencies, vegetarians should eat more vitamin B-12 and vitamin D rich foods or consider taking vitamin supplements to complement their diet.

Vitamin E and smoking

Worried about secondary smoke in the workplace or at home?

A new study in *Alive* (Feb/March 1990:1) suggests that taking more vitamin E may reduce chances of lung damage.

Cigarette smoke creates free radicals, which are tiny particles that can cause lung tissue damage.

The free radicals make it difficult for your lungs to turn the air you breathe into usable oxygen for the blood system. Free radical damage has been linked directly to the development of lung cancer, emphysema and chronic bronchitis.

Vitamin E helps trap these free radicals and prevents them

from harming the delicate lung tissue.

So, if you can't escape smoke from other people's cigarettes, vitamin E may be your best defense against lung disease.

But be careful! Too much vitamin E in the body can cause other serious problems.

Be sure to check with your doctor before you start taking extra vitamin E.

Vitamin C helps beat drinking problems, boosts recovery rate

People with an alcohol problem might help their short-term recovery by taking two grams of vitamin C a day, suggests a study reported in the June edition of the *Journal of the American College of Nutrition* (9,3:185).

Studies about alcohol detoxification—"drying out"—show that taking large doses of vitamin C really helps in clearing alcohol out of a person's system quickly.

In an experiment with 111 New York City alcoholics, three out of four of those who completed a year-long program centered around taking extra vitamins and minerals stayed sober. Regular non-nutritional therapy produces much lower success rates, reports *Men's Health* newsletter (6,8:12).

A Special Amino Acid and Vitamin Enteral (SAAVE) supplement seemed to help keep twice as many alcohol abusers in a sobriety program in California, says the manufacturer, Matrix Technologies, Inc. The findings were reported in the *Journal of Psychoactive Drugs* (1990; 22:173), says the article.

The studies are adding up: special medically-supervised diets that emphasize balanced nutrition dramatically improve chances for long-term recovery from heavy drinking.

The Recommended Dietary Allowance for vitamin C is 60

milligrams a day for people over 50. Check with your doctor before taking supplements.

Boost immune response with more vitamin C

Taking a 1,000-milligram tablet of vitamin C increases body temperature, quickly floods the bloodstream with the nutrient and seems to boost the immune system's resistance to infections.

So indicates an Arizona State University study in the April issue of the *Journal of the American College of Nutrition* (9,2:150).

Turning up the heat is one way the body fights invading disease germs.

That heat rise triggered by the big dose might be why vitamin C seems to protect some people from the common cold, suggests researcher Carol S. Johnston.

In the study, healthy men and women took by mouth one daily tablet of the sodium ascorbate form of vitamin C, the equivalent of 17 times the RDA.

Besides raising their body temperatures, the big dose also lowered the concentration of iron in their blood.

While that sounds bad, it's actually not, since germs multiply more slowly with lowered iron levels.

The raised temperatures and lowered iron levels happened only when the people took that single large daily dose of vitamin C.

The same beneficial effects probably wouldn't happen if they simply took regular vitamin-mineral supplements every day, the report suggests.

That implies that you might be better off avoiding vitamin C in supplement form until you feel a cold or other infection coming on.

In any event, don't take supplements or megadoses of any

nutrient without checking with your doctor first.

You can get the regular RDA of vitamin C in its natural form by eating at least two servings a day of citrus fruits, broccoli, Brussels sprouts, strawberries, cantaloupe and dark-green, leafy vegetables.

■ A new role for vitamin C might be in fighting cholesterol plaque build-up in arteries, suggests a study reported in the Aug. 9, 1990 edition of *Medical Tribune* (31,16:14).

Vitamin C stays on the job far longer than vitamin E in fighting oxidation of low-density lipoprotein (the "bad" LDL form of cholesterol).

University of Texas researchers believe oxidized LDL triggers atherosclerosis, or hardening of the arteries.

Because vitamin C does such a good job of battling this cholesterol, Dr. Ishwarlal Jialal suggests that the RDA should be doubled, from 60 milligrams to 120, the article says.

Hardening of the arteries causes heart disease and some strokes.

■ Vitamin C's best-known prevention role probably is its ability to neutralize several cancer-causing chemicals in cooked and processed foods.

It also acts as an antioxidant against so-called free radicals, tissue-harming substances brought into the bloodstream by food, air pollution and tobacco smoke.

Women's 2 vitamin deficiencies masquerade as deadly leukemia

Under the doctor's microscope, the abnormal blood cells seemed to shout one dreaded diagnosis — cancer of the blood, leukemia!

But in two cases, looks were deceiving, even to trained

scientists, reports the *British Medical Journal* (300,6734:1263).

After a bone biopsy in one case showed additional leukemia-like cells, doctors at Hammersmith Hospital in London even ordered an intravenous (IV) needle inserted to start chemotherapy.

The 43-year-old woman escaped unnecessary medication when late-arriving blood tests showed she had a severe shortage of vitamin B12 (also known as cobalamin).

That shortage apparently caused pernicious anemia (a lack of nutrient-carrying red blood cells), which also was successfully treated with shots of extra vitamin B12.

Another woman, 52, likewise had abnormal blood and bone-marrow cells, similar to leukemia.

It turned out that she had a shortage of another B-complex vitamin, folate (known to a few people as vitamin B9; another form is folic acid or folacin).

Her anemia also was cured by taking extra folate.

In both cases, after the women got the needed vitamins, their blood tests returned to normal, and the leukemia-like cells disappeared.

Both women had lung or airway infections when they took the blood tests. Doctors speculate that the combination of respiratory infection and anemia might have affected the test results.

Such cases might not happen often, but they do point out the need for extra care in making medical judgments.

The Recommended Dietary Allowance for folate (folacin) is 200 micrograms for men over 51, and 180 micrograms daily for women past age 51.

Natural sources of folate include dark-green, leafy vegetables; liver; dry beans, peanuts; wheat germ and whole grains.

According to the National Research Council publication *Diet and Health* (1989; pg.67), women tend to take in less folacin daily than men do.

Heat destroys the vitamin, and folate losses caused by cooking and canning can be very high, the report says.

Vitamin B12 comes naturally only in foods of animal origin. Supplying B12 are liver, muscle meats, fish, eggs, milk and milk products.

The RDA for vitamin B12 is two micrograms for men and women over age 51.

Check with your doctor before taking either vitamin B12 or folate supplements.

Eat fresh fruits and veggies for proper balance

Some scientists have suspected that higher levels of the mineral nutrient potassium might help protect you against intestinal cancers.

Now an animal study suggests that such protection might be determined by the ratio of potassium to sodium in the body.

The higher the potassium-to-sodium ratio, the better, indicates a study in *Nutrition and Cancer* (14,2:95).

Researchers found that rats with four times as much potassium as sodium in their supplemented diets had one-eighth the number of intestinal tumors.

That was when compared with the ones fed a diet containing a potassium-sodium ratio of two-to-one, the report says.

Nutritionists recommend that you get at least 1,600 to 2,000 milligrams per day of potassium in your diet. That's not hard if you eat a lot of unprocessed fruits and vegetables and fresh meat.

Taking in more potassium than sodium also helps keep your blood pressure under control.

Getting too much potassium can be as bad as getting too little. A daily intake of around 18 grams (that's 18,000 milligrams) can cause serious heart disturbances, even cardiac arrest.

Check with your doctor before taking potassium or any kind of dietary supplements.

Help prevent loss of hearing with vitamin A

If you once prided yourself on your keen sense of hearing, but you now find yourself asking people to repeat things, you may need more vitamin A in your diet.

Some cases of hearing loss may be linked to a vitamin A deficiency, *The Journal of Nutrition* (120,7:726) reports.

Studies show that a lack of vitamin A in the diet first increases the ear's sensitivity to sound. In other words, your hearing is actually better at first.

However, an increased sensitivity to noise increases the chances of noise-induced hearing loss. The very-sensitive ear can be damaged more easily and quickly than a normal ear.

So, the vitamin A deficiency does not actually cause the hearing loss. It simply makes the ear more sensitive to sound — which increases the chances of hearing loss due to noise damage.

If you suspect you may have a problem with your hearing, talk to your doctor immediately. He can help you determine whether you need more vitamin A in your diet.

Vitamin E helps protect arteries from hardening

Vitamin E may be helpful in protecting you from atherosclerosis (hardening of the arteries), says a report in the Sept. 20, 1990 *Medical Tribune* (31,19:11).

Vitamin E works as an "antioxidant" in the cells of your body. This means that it prevents oxygen molecules from combining with parts of the cell that would result in dangerous products.

For example, LDL cholesterol molecules occasionally combine with oxygen molecules to create "oxidized LDLs." These oxidized LDLs seem to damage cells, and scientists suspect that they may be one of the root causes of atherosclerosis.

Vitamin E functions as an antioxidant and prevents the LDLs from becoming oxidized. This protects the cells from damage and helps prevent atherosclerosis.

Researchers suggest that dietary antioxidants such as vitamin E could be a vital part of the treatment strategies for people with atherosclerosis as well as a good protection device for people seeking to avoid the disease.

Can vitamins help slow the aging process?

Can vitamin supplements actually help improve the immune system and delay the aging process? Scientists now think it may be possible.

Vitamin supplements may help strengthen the immune system in elderly people, suggests a study in the August 1990 *Journal of the American College of Nutrition* (9,4:363).

Maintaining a proper balance and amount of vitamins is crucial in helping the body ward off illnesses quickly and effectively. However, the study shows that most elderly people frequently have low levels of important vitamins in their bodies.

Unfortunately, this shortage of important vitamins often results in a sluggish immune system that has great trouble fighting off sicknesses. So, many elderly people suffer needlessly from common illnesses simply because their immune systems have slowed down.

Many elderly people eat very well-balanced meals, but they

still suffer from vitamin deficiencies. This is because the other medications they take often "block" the vitamins in the food from being absorbed and used in the body.

So, scientists are suggesting that elderly people talk to their physicians about vitamin supplementation. The vitamin supplement will help bring the level of vitamins in the body up to the proper level and help the immune system function as effectively as possible.

Beta carotene helps cut heart problems in half

Yellow may be the color of a healthy heart.

Yellow, that is, in the form of beta carotene, also known as previtamin A, the nutrient that gives the yellow color to carrots and squash.

Taking a 50-milligram dose of beta carotene every other day for six years seemed to help slow artery clogging in male doctors who already had heart disease, according to the Nov. 17, 1990 *Science News* (138,20:308).

Compared to men who took placebo (fake) pills, the beta carotene group had half as many "major cardiovascular events," such as heart attack or stroke, during the long-term study, according to another report of the Harvard Medical School findings in the Nov. 29, 1990 *Medical Tribune* (31,24:2).

Researchers took into account that the beta carotene men also were taking aspirin on alternate days. The 333 randomly selected participants were drawn from the much larger Physicians' Health Study. This is the study that already has produced the discovery that an aspirin every other day protects against heart attacks.

Doctors still can't say whether otherwise healthy people

would reap a heart benefit from taking beta carotene.

About 11,000 men in the large study have been taking the previtamin A supplements. Final results will be available in about four years.

Scientists guess that beta carotene hinders the formation of a harmful kind of low-density lipoprotein (LDL) cholesterol. LDL cholesterol is known as "bad" cholesterol because of the damage it sometimes does to arteries.

Once linked with oxygen in the bloodstream, the harmful kind of LDL cholesterol probably damages artery walls, leading to plaque build-up.

Like sticky putty in a pipe, the plaque deposits choke off blood flow in arteries, resulting in heart attacks and strokes.

Beta carotene, they speculate, apparently derails that process in some way.

The beta form of carotene is just one of nearly 500 carotenoid compounds occurring naturally in vegetables and fruits. The various carotenes are responsible for the yellows, oranges and reds in carrots, mangoes, papayas and apricots.

Besides those foods, other natural sources of beta carotene include broccoli, winter squash, asparagus, spinach, sweet potatoes and cantaloupe.

Beta carotene is known as previtamin A because the body converts it into active vitamin A. Vitamin A, like other fat-soluble vitamins, is stored in the body. It's easy to overdose on vitamin A.

On the other hand, it's hard to get too much beta carotene, since the body converts to vitamin form only what it needs, disposing of any excess beta carotene.

About the only bad side effect of even huge doses of beta carotene is a yellow tinged skin. But even that disappears when the beta carotene intake is reduced to normal levels.

The Recommended Dietary Allowance (RDA) for vitamin A for men over 50 is 1,000 micrograms, or one milligram, daily. For women over 50, it's 800 micrograms.

A lot of your daily vitamin A comes in the "preformed" version in foods, ready to be used and stored by the body immediately, without conversion.

If you got your RDA of vitamin A strictly from beta carotene, you would need to take in from four to six milligrams of beta carotene daily.

For example, a half cup of cooked carrots contains nearly 12 milligrams of carotene, mostly the beta type.

The 50 milligrams of beta carotene taken daily by the members of the study group is about four times the amount normally found in a half cup of carrots.

The daily study supplement was well within the "safe" range, the *SN* report noted.

However, it's best to check with your doctor before taking supplements of beta carotene or any other nutrient.

Vitamin E helps restore muscles to healthy state after exercise

If you exercise regularly, you probably need to eat more green leafy vegetables and more apples and apricots.

These foods contain large amounts of vitamin E, and studies suggest that people who exercise regularly need more vitamin E than those who do not exercise with any regularity, reports the October 1990 *Nutrition Today* (25,5 :5).

Due to the muscular stress that accompanies many types of exercise, most people experience slight muscle damage during exercise.

Based on recent studies, researchers report that vitamin E helps minimize tissue damage that could be caused by exercise and then helps restore muscles to a healthy state after exercise.

If you exercise regularly, talk to your doctor about your daily intake of vitamin E. He can advise you on how much vitamin E you should be taking in daily to minimize muscular damage and maximize the benefits of your exercise.

Vitamin E: who, what, where, why and how much?

Sources: Green leafy vegetables, shrimp and other seafood, margarine, nuts, vegetable oils, apples, apricots, peaches, wheat germ and whole-wheat flour.

Function: Promotes normal growth and development; helps reduce tissue damage after exercise; helps prevent atherosclerosis; acts as an anti-clotting agent in the blood; helps protect blood cells from oxidation (cell damage).

Who needs more of it: People over the age of 55; those who exercise regularly; people with hyperthyroidism; those with alcohol or other drug abuse.

Deficiency: Anemia, inability to concentrate, muscle weakness or damage, irritability, lack of energy and vitality, decreased sexual performance.

Too much: Possible increase in level of cholesterol in the blood; increased chance of blood clots; impairs sexual function; changes immune system responses, higher death rates.

Recommended daily allowance: Men over age 50 need 10 milligrams daily; women over age 50 need 8 milligrams daily.

Source: November 1990 FDA Consumer (24,9:31)

Weight Loss

Easy 'OJ diet' might help you lose weight

You don't need to send off for it if you see an ad for an "orange juice diet."

That's because you've got the whole diet right in your supermarket produce section or chilled juice case.

It's simple: scientists have discovered that water mixed with fructose suppresses your appetite better than glucose with water or even diet drinks. Fructose is the kind of sugar found in fruits.

Drink a glass of fructose-rich orange juice a half hour to one hour before a meal, the results suggest.

You'll eat fewer calories during the next meal and still feel comfortably full, indicates a Yale University researcher in the *American Journal of Clinical Nutrition* (51,3:428).

The diet drink, glucose-water and fructose-rich fruit juice all seem to work as appetite suppressants.

It's just that fructose worked better than sugar-water. And, the glucose-water worked better than drinks flavored with the low-calorie sweetener aspartame (brand names NutraSweet and Equal).

Plain water was least effective of the four.

In the fructose part of the study, overweight men ate nearly 300 fewer calories at lunch. Overweight women consumed an average of 431 fewer mid-day calories.

Their intakes were compared with similarly overweight men and women who drank plain water before lunch.

Even when the participants switched drinks, the results were the same. The new ones drinking the fructose-sweetened lemonade mixture ate fewer calories than those drinking the other lemonade-flavored mixtures.

But what about the calories in the fructose drink itself? You might well ask.

Since the fructose drink was about 200 calories, the net calorie suppression was about 100 to 230 calories per meal.

That still puts the orange juice diet ahead of its glucose, aspartame and plain water competition.

If only for one meal, that still adds up to a savings of 700 calories a week or 36,400 calories a year, certainly enough to make a difference over the long run.

Long-term, slow weight loss is the healthiest form of weight loss for most people.

The diet benefit, however, doesn't carry over to soft drinks sweetened with high-fructose corn syrup. People who drank a lot of aspartame-sweetened diet drinks reduced their intake of calories from sugar more than those who gulped regular soda pop, says a report three months later in the same journal (51,6:963).

Lose weight to help keep your liver in good health

Losing weight may help your heart — and your liver, researchers report in *Science News* (135,21:332).

If you're at least 11 percent over your ideal weight, you may be headed for liver disease. Thirty-nine people who enrolled in a New York City study were.

Researchers put those 39 people on a diet and exercise program. Eighteen months later, 17 people had lost 10 percent of their body weight and showed no signs of liver disease.

Those who couldn't stick to the program or gained weight continued to have liver problems.

You could call the liver the chemical factory of the body. It's the largest gland in the body, and it stores bile, a substance which helps digest food. The liver also filters wastes and toxins from the blood, such as drugs, bacteria and food additives.

It also stores vitamins and minerals such as iron, which is important for the production of healthy red blood cells.

When the liver stops working, the body is in trouble. Unfortunately, liver disease often produces no symptoms, so it is hard to diagnose.

One of the earliest symptoms is jaundice, which causes the skin to turn yellow.

Jaundice results when the liver fails to filter certain substances from the blood — a sign that the liver system is breaking down.

If you are overweight, you may want to check with your doctor about starting a safe and healthy diet and exercise program to help reduce your risk of liver disease.

After all, the best way to fight liver disease is to prevent it.

More to lose than weight

Scientists have found a new weight-loss incentive for all those would-be dieters who haven't gotten serious about their diets yet.

The results of a recent study reported in *The New England*

Journal of Medicine (322,13:882) suggest that all women who are mildly to moderately overweight have a risk of heart disease 80 percent higher than women who maintain their ideal body weight.

Weight gain during adulthood increases the risk of coronary disease. And the older you get, the greater your risk becomes.

These results indicate that being overweight is a major cause of death from heart disease among women in the United States.

Bouts with gout

People who are overweight might greatly reduce their chances of suffering from gout by losing weight — but only if they lose weight slowly.

Rapid weight loss can actually increase your chances of getting gout.

A sensible diet that helps you lose weight slowly is much more effective in preventing gout than a crash diet, suggests a report in the *Harvard Medical School Health Letter* (14,6:1).

You also can help prevent gout by avoiding some foods that seem to trigger bouts with gout: anchovies, asparagus, brains, kidney, liver, mincemeats, mushrooms, sardines and sweet-breads.

Caffeine and alcohol intake should be limited as well.

Diet-and-exercise teamwork

Ever wonder why exercise helps you lose weight faster? *Stay Healthy* (3,12:46) has the answer:

Dieting lowers your metabolic rate, or the rate at which you burn off calories, and exercise boosts your metabolic rate back to normal. Thirty minutes of daily exercise can burn off 150 to 200 extra calories a day.

And here's more good news from *Good Health Bulletin* (II,3:2): regular exercise also keeps your heart healthy by producing an enzyme that breaks down fats in the bloodstream.

Exercise helps you maintain, not lose weight

You've just started a new exercise program and are excited because the exercise is going to help you lose weight, right?

Well, researchers have added a new twist to that theory.

According to a July report in *The Physician and Sportsmedicine* (18,7:113), exercise is not a big help in losing weight—you would have to walk about 22 miles to lose one pound.

However, exercise is extremely helpful in helping you keep the weight off once you've lost it through eating less.

Exercise should be viewed as a "weight-maintenance tool" rather than a weight-loss tool.

It is fairly common for people who have lost some weight to gain it back simply because they didn't begin an exercise maintenance program.

On the other hand, those who commit themselves to an exercise program after their weight-loss program are usually successful in keeping the old pounds off.

Being too thin may shorten your life span

Being thin is not as in vogue as it used to be, especially if you are between the ages of 55 and 74, says the *Archives of Internal Medicine* (150,5:1065). Apparently, it is better for elderly people to carry a few extra pounds rather than be underweight.

Researchers are finding that older skinny people are up to 1.6 times more likely to die than medium or over-weight people.

Being overweight caused more problems than being too thin only when the extra weight complicated high blood pressure or diabetes (two weight-related conditions).

When are you too thin?

Researchers from this study defined the average height for men to be 5 feet 9 inches and the average height for women to be 5 feet 4 inches.

"Thin" men weighed under 149 pounds, and "thin" women weighed under 126 pounds.

Ask your doctor to help you determine your ideal and healthiest weight.

Help reverse drug-induced impotence by losing weight

Many men who take diuretics or "water pills" to help control their hypertension suffer from a physically and psychologically unpleasant side effect — sexual impotence.

But scientists may have discovered a way to reverse this aggravating side effect.

Moderate weight loss may help reverse this drug-induced sexual problem, suggests a report in the Sept. 22, 1990 *Science News* (138,12:189).

In the recent study, 35 men who suffered from drug-induced impotence went on diets and lost an average of about 10 pounds each.

All but three of the men who lost the weight reported obvious improvement in erectile ability.

In other words, 90 percent of the men in the study who lost weight experienced relief from the drug-induced sexual impotence.

Researchers suggest that men who suffer from drug-induced impotence should talk with their physicians.

The doctor can prescribe a safe diet that will help the men control their hypertension as well as lose weight to reverse the drug side effects.

Raise resting metabolism rate with exercise

You've argued with your conscience about it before.

You know you need to lose some weight, but you're afraid to diet because dieting is supposed to lower your metabolism so much that you gain all the weight back.

It's a legitimate fear. But now that fear appears to be unfounded.

Until now, scientists have thought that people who lose weight through low-calorie diets ended up in a catch-22 situation: losing weight slows down the body's resting metabolic rate. Your resting metabolic rate is the amount of energy needed to maintain basic body functions, such as breathing and heart beat.

A slower metabolic rate is your body's way of coping with less food. It helps the body function normally with a smaller amount of food. The problem is that a slower metabolism makes it easier to gain weight and harder to keep off those unwanted pounds.

Since your body only needs a small amount of food to function, the excess calories are transformed into weight gain.

However, studies now are showing that exercise can help restore a healthy metabolism, says the Aug. 8, 1990 *The Journal of the American Medical Association* (264,6:707).

Apparently, people who lose weight by combining a low-calorie diet and exercise will experience a drop in their metabolism at first. In fact, the exercise may even increase the initial drop.

However, after a few weeks of this routine, the metabolism springs back to a level that is normal for their new, lower body weight.

The new metabolism will be slightly slower than the original metabolism. However, the new metabolic rate is perfect for the new body weight.

So, dieters should not be concerned about a plunging metabolic rate. As long as you exercise, your metabolic rate will spring back up to a healthy level that will suit your new, thinner body.

Index

A

Acarosan 47
Acetaminophen 124
Acetazolamide 129
Acne problems 167
Acrodynia 176
Aerobic exercise 136
Aerobics
  arthritis 9
Age-related macular degen-
  eration (AMD) 148
Aging 1, 3
  and dry skin 232
Aging process
  immune system
    vitamins 285
Agitation 120

Air pollution
  free radicals
    vitamins 281
Alcohol 124
  dry skin 222
  insomnia 237
  osteoporosis risk 215
  detoxification
    vitamin C 278
  effects on psoriasis 227
  gout 294
  polycythemia vera 265
  sleep apnea 242
  vitamin E 288
Alcohol intake 49
Alcoholism
  and pain relievers 124

Alka-Seltzer Plus Night-
Time Cold
Medicine   111
Allergens   43
Allergic reaction
anaphylaxis   230
bee/insect stings   229
contact dermatitis   224
Allergies   59, 120
cat allergies   59
dust mites   46
house dust   45
molds   46
pollen allergies
allergic symptoms   43
radioallergosorbent
testing   44
tannic acid   59
Alstroemeria
South American lily
poisonous plants   231
Aluminum   133
pots and pans   177
Alzheimer's
disease   7, 8,
153, 209
aluminum pots and
pans   177
aspirin therapy   8
memory loss   7
nerve growth factor   7
sleep apnea   240
sleepwalkers
Seasonal Affective
Disorder   219
Amalgam   173

Amalgam fillings
alternatives to Amalgam
fillings   174
American Heart Associa-
tion   269
American Sleep Disorder
Association   236
Amino acid   269
hyperhomo-
cysteinemia   269
methionine   270
Amsler grid   148
Anacin-3   124
Anaphylaxis
insect stings   230
Anemia   52
false hemoglobin   52
vitamin B12 defi-
ciency   281
vitamin E   288
Angina   58
Animal-transmitted dis-
eases
symptoms   159
Antacids   119
and magnesium   134
and sodium-bicarbon-
ate   134
contain aluminum   133
Anti-aging pill   4
Anti-arrhythmic
drugs   117
Anti-baldness drug   123
minoxidil   123
Anti-ulcer drug   126
Anti-ulcer medication
misoprostol   126

Antibiotics
  quinine 166
Antibodies 44
Antidepressants 104
  imipramine 104
Antihistamines 110
  and drowsiness 110
  contact dermatitis 225
  diphenhydramine 110
  sedative types 111
  triprolidine 111
Antioxidants 150. *See
  also Vitamins*
  effects on cancer 31
  vitamin C 280
  vitamin E
    prevents athero-
    sclerosis 284
  vitamin E and sele-
    nium 274
Anxiety
  and insomnia 235
  sleeping problems
    sleeping pills 238
Appetite suppressant
  and fruit juices 168
  orange juice diet 291
Apple-cider vinegar
  vinegar test
    vitamins and
    minerals 275
Arrhythmia 117
Arteries 24
  beta carotene
    prevents clogging 286
  brain blood supply
    dietary salt 266

cholesterol build-up
  vitamin C 280
hardening 24
  vitamin B 269
  vitamin C 280
  vitamin E 284
Arteries, hardening of
  vitamin E 267
Artery walls
  dietary salt 266
Arthritis 9, 10, 11, 12,
  13, 15, 17, 122, 162
  canes 12
  cold therapy 15
  exercise 9, 11, 14
    aerobic exercise 13
    swimming 11
    two-hour rule 10
    walking, skating, skiing
    and cycling 10
  fish oil 17
  heat therapy 15
  hormone
    interleukin-1 18
  joint pain
    exercise 9
  massage 12
  omega-3 fatty acids 17
  rheumatoid arthritis 8
  safety devices 12
  walkers 12
  walking 12
  weight lifting 3
Arthritis Foundation 12
Artificial light
  Seasonal Affective Disor-
    der 218

Artificial sweeteners
aspartame 292
Ascorbic acid 134
Aspartame
NutraSweet 291
orange juice diet
weight loss 291
Equal 291
Aspirin 96, 119, 226
and migraine head-
aches 155
crushed in lotion
for shingles pain 226
disoriented 122
dizziness 122
heart problems
and beta carotene 285
salicylism 122
Aspirin therapy 8
heart attacks 246
migraine headaches 178
migraine pain 246
rheumatoid arthritis 8
Asthma 47, 99. See also
Breathing problems
selenium defi-
ciency 272, 274
Atenolol 116
Atherosclero-
sis 186, 189, 207, 269
and vitamin E 267
hyperhomocysteinemia 269
vitamin B 269
vitamin C 280
vitamin E 284, 288
Athlete's foot medicine
contact dermatitis 226
Ativan 103

Atrial fibrillation
risk of stroke
aspirin therapy 245
Attention lapse
sleeping problems 238
Azotemia 123

B

Babesiosis 165
Bacteria
and urinary tract infec-
tions 253
liver filters 293
Bathing
and insomnia 236
Baths, bubble
and urinary tract infec-
tions 254
Benadryl 111
Benzodiazepine 103
and broken hip 103
Beta-blocker 22
Beta-carotene 83
heart problems 286
sources of 287
tinged skin 286
Beta-glucans 201
Bicycling
stationary 22
Bile
liver
weight loss 293
Biotin 270
Bladder cancer
selenium
deficiency 273. See
also Cancer

Bleeding ulcers   126. *See also Ulcers*
Blindness   161, 174
Blisters   16
Blocked blood vessels   124
Blood
  anemia   281
  anti-clotting drugs
    anti-stroke
    therapy   246
  clotting
    vitamin E   288
  leukemia
    vitamin deficiency   281
  pernicious anemia
    vitamin B12 defi-
    ciency   281
  plasma
    selenium defi-
    ciency   274
  Raynaud's disease   265
Blood cells
  polycythemia vera   264
Blood cholesterol   169. *See also Cholesterol*
Blood clot   48, 135
  cholesterol   263
  phlebitis   261
  tissue plasminogen
    activator   263
  vitamin B
    hyperhomo-
    cysteinemia   269
  vitamin E   289
Blood disorder
  polycythemia vera   264

Blood flow
  in arteries
    beta carotene   286
Blood Pressure   19
Blood pres-
    sure   1, 3, 24, 91, 109
  blood fibrin level   263
  diastolic   23
  diastolic level   116
  exercise   22
  high blood pres-
    sure   1, 19, 21
  hypertension
    sexual impotence   296
  job demands   25
  salt, dietary   266
  systolic   23
  vitamin C   19
  weight loss   22
    risk of being too
    thin   296
Blood sugar   90
Bloodshot eyes
  polycythemia vera   265
Bloodstream
  immune system
    vitamin C   279
  vitamins and minerals
    absorption into   276
Body clock
  shift workers   243
Body rhythms   37
  effects on immune sys-
    tem   37
Body temperature
  immune system
    vitamin C   279

Bone biopsy
  leukemia
    vitamin deficiency 281
Bone disease 81. *See also*
    Osteoporosis
  brittle bone disease
    osteoporosis 1
Bone-marrow cells
  leukemia 281
Borrelia burgdorferi 162
Brain damage 174
Brain disease 48
Breast cancer 37, 64,
    186. *See also Cancer*
Breast vascular conges-
    tion 125
Breathing
  metabolic rate 298
Breathing problems
  airway infections 281
  asthma
    selenium defi-
    ciency 274
  bronchitis
    vitamin E 277
  emphysema
    vitamin E 277
  insect stings
    allergic reaction 229
  secondary smoke
    lung damage 278
  sleep apnea 238
  snoring 239
Breathlessness 58
British Red Cross 4
Brittle-bone
    disease 1, 170, 212. *See
    also Osteoporosis*

Broken hip 103, 202
Bronchitis 57. *See also
    Breathing problems*
  effects of salt 57
  effects of vitamin C and
    niacin 57
  secondary smoke
    vitamin E 279
Bull's eye rash 162

C

Caffeine
  and dry skin 222
  and insomnia 236
  and osteoporosis 216
  gout 294
Calcitrol
  psoriasis 230
  vitamin D3 230
Calcium 83, 133, 134,
    192, 202. *See also
    Minerals*
  absorption of
    vinegar test 275
  and osteoporosis 215
  and too much salt 211
  effects of caffeine
    osteoporosis risk 216
  menopause 81
  sources of 205
  timed-release forms 276
Calcium carbonate 79
  absorption of
    vinegar test 276
Calcium channel
    blocker 22

Calories 168
  low-calorie diet
    metabolic rate 297
  weight loss
    dieting 295
    exercise 295
    orange juice diet 291
Cancer 63, 67, 68, 105,
    124, 166, 185, 196, 204
  and garlic 188
  and low-fat milk 67
  and nails 68
  and stress 204
  and whole milk 68
  bladder
    selenium defi-
    ciency 273
  breast cancer 27, 28,
    30, 32, 35, 36, 38
    cell division cycles 38
    chemotherapy 27
    circadian sleep-wake
    cycle 38
    ductal cancer 35
    effects of cruciferous
    vegetables 28
    effects of estrogen 29
    effects of selenium 31
    effects of vitamin E 31
    hormonal treat-
    ment 36
    hormone levels 39
    lumpectomy 34
    metastatic 39
    radiation therapy 35
    radical mastectomy 34
    surgical treatments 27
    survival rates 27

cancer risks 3
cancer-causing chemicals
  vitamin C 280
chemotherapy
  vitamin deficiency 281
chlorambucil 105
colon cancer 30, 79, 82
  barium enemas 86
  effects of milk 82
  polyps 86
colorectal cancer 81
  effects of fiber 86
  effects of potas-
  sium 82
cyclophosphamide 105
effects of spices 69
endometrial cancers 33
intestinal cancer
  effects of potas-
  sium 282
leukemia
  retinoic acid 276
  vitamin A 276
  vitamin deficiency 281
lung cancer
  secondary smoke 278
melphalan 105
premenopausal breast
  cancer 39
radiotherapy 105
rectal cancer 30, 82
selenium deficiency 272
thiotepa 105
treosulfan 105
Canes 12, 14
Capsaicin cream 172

Capsules
  vitamins and minerals
    absorption of 276
Carbamazepine
  tegretol 121
Carbon monoxide 142
Carcinogens 64, 108
Cardiac arrest
  potassium 282
Cardiac arrhythmias 142
Cardiac/nervous disor-
    ders 162
Cardiovascular dis-
    ease 137, 157, 190
Cardiovascular problems
  beta carotene 286
Carotenoid compounds
  beta carotene
    sources of 286
Carotenoids 64
Carotid arteriography 49
Carotid artery 48
Carotid atherosclerosis 48
Cast iron
  pots and pans 178
Cat scratch fever 163
Cataracts
  and milk 171
  and steroids 150
  and the sun 150
Centrax 103
Cerebral
    hemorrhage 73. *See
    also Stroke*
Chemotherapy 28, 35,
    36, 105
  and body rhythm 37

leukemia
  vitamin deficiency 281
Chest pain 10
Chewing tobacco 154
Chicken pox
  herpes virus 226
Chlorambucil 105
Cholesterol 22, 24, 71,
    72, 75, 76, 157, 169,
    183, 186, 189, 199, 203,
    204, 269
  and heart disease 185
  and whole milk 68
  blood clots 263
  effects of oatrim 201
  effects of potassium 26
  effects of psyllium 77
  HDL 23, 76, 143, 196
  LDL 22, 74, 77, 199
    niacin 272
    vitamin C and E 280
    vitamin E 284
  niacin 271, 272
  polyunsaturated fatty
    acids 74
  vitamin C 280
  vitamin E 289
  when levels are too
    low 73
Choline 209
Chromium 74, 90
  sources of 75
Chromium picolinate 74
Chronic bronchitis 53
Chronic fatigue syn-
    drome 145
Chronobiology 37

Cigarettes
  secondary smoke
    vitamin E   278
Circadian rhythm
  body clock
    sleeping problems   243
  depression
    Seasonal Affective
    Disorder   218
Cirrhosis   208
Clogged arteries   184. *See
    also Arteries*
Clonidine
  stroke medication   247
Cobalamin
  deficiency of
    leukemia   281
Coffee
  and osteoporosis   216
Colloidal oatmeal
  contact dermatitis   225
Cologne
  contact dermatitis   226
Colon
    cancer   64, 206. *See
    also Cancer*
  effects of calcium   79
  skin tags   85
Colonoscopy   86
Common cold
  immune system
    vitamin C   279
Condoms
  urinary tract infec-
    tions   254
Confusion   120, 171
Congestive heart fail-
    ure   117

Conjunctivitis
  bloodshot eyes
    polycythemia vera   265
Constipation   130
  and hypothyroidism   249
Contac   124
Contact
    dermatitis   224. *See
    also Skin problems*
  among the elderly   233
  common causes   225
  Nickel-based jew-
    elry   224
Contraceptive foams
  urinary tract infec-
    tions   254
Contraceptives
  contact dermatitis   226
  urinary tract infec-
    tions   253
Cookware   177
Cornea   149
Coronary arteries   186
Coronary disease
  weight loss   294
Coronary heart disease
    143, 157,
    196, 199, 203
Corticosteroids   119, 134
Cosmetics
  and dry skin   223
  contact dermatitis   224
Coughing
  stress incontinence   256
Cramping   20
Cyclophosphamide   105

D

Deafness   174
Deer tick   162
  babesiosis   165
Dehydration   153
Delirium   120
Demarest   111
Dementia   130, 153
  sleep apnea   240
Deodorants
  contact dermatitis   224
Depression   51, 104, 130
  light therapy
    SAD   217
  Seasonal Affective Disor-
    der   217
  urinary inconti-
    nence   256
Detergents
  contact dermatitis   224
Diabe-
    tes   37, 49, 89, 90, 196
  and high blood pres-
    sure   115
  blood sugar   90
  blood sugar disorder   89
  fructan   93
  fructose   90
  glucose   90
  glucose intolerant   90
  low insulin index   116
  niacin   272
  non-insulin-depen-
    dent   90
  protein and kidney
    damage   197
  sources of chromium   90
  Type II   90, 91
  weight loss   296
Diabetes mellitus   222
Diabetic neuropathy   172
Diallyl sulfide   67
Diaphragms
  urinary tract infec-
    tions   253
Diarrhea   20, 95, 98,
  126, 130
  selenium   275
Diet   37
  and colon cancer   206
  and magnesium   186
  choline   209
  chromium and diabe-
    tes   90
  colon and rectal can-
    cers   83
  crash diet
    gout   294
  cruciferous veg-
    etables   201
  effects of a restricted
    diet   198
  effects of basil   206
  effects of beans and peas
    on cancer   87
  effects of fiber   86
  effects of ginger   97
  effects of olive oil   189
  effects of salt   57
  effects on Chronic fatigue
    syndrome   145
  fat   206
  fat content
    and heart disease   203

fatty acids
  completely hydroge-
    nated 208
  partially hydroge-
    nated 208
  unsaturated 208
fiber 124
fish and heart at-
  tacks 184
food and medica-
  tions 114
garlic
  and heart attacks 188
hearing loss 169
high-fat diets
  effects on breast can-
    cer 32
high-fiber 33
high-fiber cereals 71
high-sugar 31
low cholesterol
  and heart disease 187
low-fat
  and heart disease 199
  and immune sys-
    tem 193
low-fat milk
  effects on cancer 67
low-protein
  and kidney dam-
    age 197
low-salt 24
low-sugar
  effects on cancer 30
microwaved food 108
monounsaturated fatty
  acids 189

orange juice
  weight loss 291
phenols
  sources of phenols 63
polyunsaturated fatty
  acids 74
poor nutrition
  weakened bones 202
raw vegetables
  effects on choles-
    terol 201
salt 82
saturated
  fats 74, 84, 157, 189
  effects on cancer 32
sources of chromium 90
starches 84
stress diet 205
too much salt
  brain tissue dam-
    age 266
  loss of calcium 211
trans fatty acids 207
vegetarian
  vitamin deficien-
    cies 277
weight loss
  liver health 293
  metabolic rate 294
  orange juice diet 291
  sexual impotence 296
Dieting 168
Digestive problems 95
diarrhea
  selenium 275
selenium deficiency 272
Diltiazem hydrochlo-
  ride 22

Diphenhydramine 110
Dish-washing soaps
  contact dermatitis 224
Disoriented 122, 153
Diuretics
  sexual impotence
    weight loss 296
  water pills
    sexual impotence 296
Dizziness 10, 122, 144
Douching 156
  contact dermatitis 226
  infections 156
Drug abuse
  vitamin E 288
Drug interactions 130
Drug side effects
  sexual impotence
    weight loss 296
Drugs
  and insomnia 237. *See also Generic brand drugs*
  and nutrition 133
  beta-blocker
    propranolol hydrochloride 22
  diltiazem hydrochloride 22
  diuretics
    sexual impotence 296
  impotence
    weight loss 296
  liver filters 293
  stroke recovery inhibition 247
  water pills
    sexual impotence 296

Dry mouth 120, 154
Dry skin 221. *See also Skin problems*
  moisturizing lotions 222
  soaps 232
Dust mites 46
  acarosan 47

E

Ear
  hearing loss
    vitamin A
      deficiency 283
Ear crease 181
Electric blankets
  effects on cancer 41
  electromagnetic
    fields 41
Ellagic acid 64
  sources of 64
Emphysema 53. *See also Breathing problems*
  secondary smoke
    vitamin E 277
Endometrial
  cancer 186. *See also Cancer*
Energy
  lack of
    vitamin E 288
  metabolic rate
    dieting 297
    exercise 297
Energy loss
  sleeping problems
    skimping on sleep 238

Enzyme
  glutathione peroxidase
    selenium defi-
    ciency 274
Epileptic seizures 121
Equal
  orange juice diet
    weight loss 291
Erratic heart rhythm 104
Estrogen 29, 37
  and cholesterol 185
  and heart disease 185
Estrogen replacement
  therapy 185
Estrogen-blocker
  indole-3-carbinol 29
Etidronate
  and osteoporosis 214
Excedrin PM 111
Exercise 2, 9, 11, 14,
    22, 37, 49
  aerobic exercise 13, 22
  and air pollutants 143
  and colorectal can-
    cers 83
  and fitness 135
  and heart attack 135
  and heart problems 187
  and insomnia 236
  and irregular heart-
    beats 142
  blood pressure 264
  calories
    metabolic rate 295
  chest pain 10
  dangers of 143
  decreases fibrin
    levels 263

  dissolve blood clots 263
  dizziness 10
  faintness 10
  for Chronic Fatigue
    Syndrome 145
  high-density lipopro-
    tein 136
  lack of
    blood clots 261
  lower blood pres-
    sure 136
  maintain weight
    loss 295
  nausea 10
  phlebitis 262
  pulse 14
  sleep apnea 241
  swimming 11
  target heart rate 13
  two-hour rule 10
  vitamin E 288
  weight loss 295
    liver health 293
    metabolic rate 295
Eye problems
  age-related macular
    degeneration
    (AMD) 148
  effects of caffeine 147
  Pseudomonas aeruginos
    bacteria 149
  "wet" AMD 148
Eyedrop drug therapy 151
Eyes
  cataracts
    and milk 171
  macula 148
Eyesight 147

F

Face creams
contact dermatitis 226
Faintness 10
Fat 33
body fat
effects on breast cancer 36
effects on cancer 33
saturated 275
upper-body fat 36
Fatigue
polycythemia vera 265
selenium 274
sleeping problems
skimping on sleep 238
Fatty deposits 200
Fever 176
Fiber 30, 33, 124, 183, 204
and heart attacks 184
cancer protection 30
effects on cancer 33
Fibrin
blood clots 263
heart disease 263
Fish oil 17, 169, 184, 195, 197
and gallstones 195
heartburn 197
Fitness 9. *See also Exercise*
Flat feet 141
Flea wort 204
Flu 97
Fluoride 133
and osteoporosis 215

Fluoxetine 104
Folate 192. *See also Vitamins*
deficiency of folate
and leukemia 281
natural sources of 282
vegetarian diet 277
Folic acid 133, 134
Food
and medicines 170
dairy products
and cataracts 171
galactose 171
iodine content 167
Foot ulcers 89
and smoking 89
and vascular disease 89
Fountain of Youth
hormone 3
Free radicals
antioxidant
vitamin C 280
secondary smoke
lung damage 278
Fructan 93
Fructose 90, 168
orange juice diet
weight loss 291
Functional incontinence
symptoms of 257
Fungus 161
spores 46

G

Galactose 171
Gallbladder disease 37
Gallstones 195

Gardeners
  poisonous plants 231
Garlic 188
  and cancer 188
  and heart attacks 188
  effects on cancer 67
Gastroesophageal re-
    flux 98
Gastrointestinal diseases
  and skimping on
      sleep 239. *See also*
      Digestive problems
Gastrointestinal distur-
      bances 119
  corticosteroids 119
Generic brand drugs 113
Genetic disorder
  phytosterolemia 124
Germs
  immune system
      vitamin C 279
Ginger 97
Gland
  liver
      weight loss 293
Glaucoma 106, 147,
    151. *See also Eyes*
  and taste distur-
      bances 128
  effects of caffeine 147
  problems with eye
      drops 106
  side effects of medica-
      tion 106
  timolol 152
Glucose 90, 168
  orange juice diet
      weight loss 291

Glucose intolerant 90
Glutathione peroxidase
  selenium deficiency 274
Gout 20
  foods that trigger 294
  weight loss 294
Gum disease 170
  and osteoporosis 215

H

Hair loss
  selenium 275
Hair spray
  contact dermatitis 225
Hair-care products
  contact dermatitis 225
Haloperidol
  stroke medication
      inhibits recovery 247
Hardened arteries 124.
      See also Atherosclerosis
Hay-fever 119
Headaches 172
Health Tips 153
Hearing loss 169
  noise-induced
      vitamin A defi-
          ciency 283
Heart 9, 142
  and snacking 183
  effects of potassium 25
  enlarged heart 188
  fluttering
      risk of stroke 245
  heart disease
      exercise 2
  heart medication
      (A.C.E.) inhibitor 107

irregular heart
 rhythms 196
medications
 irregular heart-
 beat 117
weight loss 293
Heart attack 50, 58, 74,
 76, 99, 104, 156, 184
 and ear crease 181
 aspirin therapy 246
 beta carotene 286
 polycythemia vera 265
 risks of heart attack 36
 vitamin B 270
Heart beat
 metabolic rate 298
Heart block 104
Heart damage 49
Heart disease 25, 54, 72,
 76, 81, 99, 124, 155, 157,
 167, 182, 186, 203
 and caffeine 110
 and estrogen 185
 and fibrin 263
 and low-fat diet 199
 atherosclerosis
 vitamin C 280
 effects of garlic 76
 risk of
 weight loss 294
 weight loss 294
Heart problems 181
 and exercise 187
 beta carotene 286
 left ventricular hypertrophy (LVH) 188
 potassium 283

propranolol
 side effects 114
 selenium deficiency 273
 skimping on sleep 238
Heart rate 176
Heart-rhythm 99
Heartburn 98
 and asthma 99
 esophagus 98
 gastroesophageal re-
 flux 98
 natural remedies 99
Helicobacter pylori bacteria 100
Hemoglobin 52
Hemorrhagic stroke 74
Hemorrhoid products
 contact dermatitis 226
Herbal medicines 155
Herbicide
 poisonous plants 228
Herbs
 feverfew 155
Hernia 2
Herpes virus
 shingles
 pain relief 226
High blood pressure 25,
 37, 49, 57, 73, 81,
 91, 115, 157, 167,
 188. *See also Blood
 pressure*
 and diabetes 115
 beta-blocker 22
 propranolol hydrochlo-
 ride 22
 calcium channel
 blocker 22

low-salt diet 24
potassium 21
High cholesterol 137. *See also Cholesterol*
High-density lipoprotein 136
Histamine 44
Histoplasmosis 60
Hormone 3, 18, 36
anti-aging pill 4
estradiol
effects on cancer 33
estrogen 29
estrone
effects on cancer 33
fountain of youth 3
human growth hormone 3
insulin 24
Hot tubs 11
and dry skin 224
and urinary tract infections 254
Human papillomavirus
wart removal
allergic reaction 231
Hydralazine 116
Hydrocortisone cream
contact
dermatitis 225, 233
Hydrogenated fats 189
Hydrogenation 207, 208
Hygiene 4
Hyperhomocysteinemia 269
Hypertension 22, 57, 91, 110, 137. *See also High blood pressure*

drug therapy
sexual impotence 296
Hyperthyroidism
vitamin E 288. *See also Thyroid problems*

I

Ibuprofen 118
and kidney function 118
Ideal weight
weight loss 293
Imipramine
side effects 104
Immune system 44, 136
aging process
vitamins 285
defective immune system 194
selenium deficiency 274
vitamin C 279
natural sources of 280
vitamin E 288
Immune system
defects 160
Immunosuppressive
therapy 160
Impotence 132
drug-induced
weight loss 296
Incontinence 132. *See also Urinary incontinence*
Indigestion 96
antacids 96
aspirin 96
effects of bananas 96
ulcer medicines 96

Indole glycosinolates   66
Indole-3-carbinol
  in cruciferous vegetables
    cancer-fighting
    effects   29
Infection   156
  immune system
    vitamin C   279
Inflammatory bowel
    disease   126
Injured ears
  exercises for dizzi-
    ness   144
Insect stings   229
Insomnia   174, 235. *See
    also Sleep problems*
  causes   235
  helpful tips   236
Insulin   24, 31, 75, 183
Integument
  skin disorders   232. *See
    also Skin problems*
Interleukin-1   18
Intestinal cancer
  potassium   282. *See also
    Cancer*
Intestinal diseases
  selenium deficiency   273
Intestinal disorders
  laxatives   95
Intestinal hemorrhages
  polycythemia vera   265
Iodine   167. *See also
    Minerals*
Iron   124, 133, 193. *See
    also Minerals*
  immune system   279

minerals
  liver   293
Irregular heart
  rhythms   142. *See
    also Heart*
Irregular heartbeats   142
Irritability
  and selenium   275
  and vitamin E   288
Itching   176. *See also Skin
    problems*
  insect stings
    allergic reactions   229
  lichen planus   231
  South American lily
    allergic reaction   231

J

Jaundice   166
  liver health
    weight loss   293
Jet lag
  and insomnia   235
  Seasonal Affective Disor-
    der   219
Jogging   13, 22, 143. *See
    also Exercise*
Joint pain   9
Joints, swollen
  insect stings
    allergic reaction   229

K

Kidney damage   122
  azotemia   123
  effects of protein   197
Kidney disease   198

Kidney failure   118, 198
Kidney stones   20
Kidneys   174
  damage to kidneys
    urinary tract infec-
      tions   256

L

Laser beam wart removal
  adverse reactions   231
Laughing
  stress incontinence   256
Laxatives   95
  diarrhea   95
  gastrointestinal tract   95
  nausea   95
  stomach cramping   95
  vomiting   95
Lecithin   209
  sources of   209
Left ventricular hypertrophy
    (LVH)   188
  and high blood pres-
    sure   188
Leg cramps   176
Legumes
  effects on cancer   33
Lesion   161
Lethargy
  polycythemia vera   265
Leukemia   105. *See also*
    Blood
  vitamin A   276
  vitamin deficiency   281
Libritabs   103
Librium   103
Lichen planus

skin problems
  and liver disease   231
Lichen simples chronicus
  skin problems   233
Licorice   167
Life span
  sleeping problems
    skimping on sleep   238
Light box
  light therapy
    Seasonal Affective
      Disorder   218
Light therapy
  Alzheimer's disease   219
  Seasonal Affective Disor-
    der
    depression   217
Limbitrol   103
Linoleic acid   65
  sources of   65
Lipstick
  contact dermatitis   226
Liver   174
  and skin problems   231
  bile
    weight loss   293
  damaged by niacin   270
  minerals
    iron   293
  weight loss   293
Liver damage
  alcohol and pain reliev-
    ers   124
Liver disease   118
Losing weight
  jogging   143

Lotion
  crushed aspirin
    shingles pain re-
    lief 226
Low blood
    pressure 104. *See
    also Blood pressure*
Lumpectomy 34, 38
Lung cancer
  free radicals 53. *See
    also Cancer*
  selenium deficiency 273
Lung damage
  secondary smoke
    vitamin E 278
Lung health 9
Lung infection 60
  histoplasmosis 60
Lyme disease
  Borrelia burgdorferi 162
  bull's eye rash 162
  symptoms of 162
Lymph glands 160

M

Macula 148
Magnesium 91, 124,
    134, 193. *See also
    Minerals*
  and high blood pres-
    sure 91
  sources of 91, 186
Maprotiline
  side effects 104
Massage 12
  sleep apnea 242
Mastectomy 38

Meals
  and insomnia 236
Medications 129
  and constipation 130
  and depression 130
  and diarrhea 130
  and digestion prob-
    lems 130
  and dry mouth 130
  and food 170
  and gastrointestinal
    irritation 130
  and impotence 132
  and incontinence 132
  and mental confu-
    sion 130
  and nutritional distur-
    bances 130
  and sense of taste 130
  sleep apnea 241
Medicine
  effectiveness 170
Melanoma 68
Melatonin 41
Melphalan 105
Memory loss 7
Menopause 32, 35
  cancer risks 32
  urinary tract infec-
    tions 253
Menrium 103
Menstrual cycle 37, 38
  immune response
    effects on breast can-
    cer 37
  immune system 39

Mental handicaps
  urinary inconti-
    nence 257
Mental sluggishness
  polycythemia vera 265
Mercury 174
Mercury poisoning
  effects of 175
Metabolic rate
  low-calorie diet
    weight loss 297
  weight loss 295
Metabolism
  weight loss 297
Methionine
  vitamin B 270
Metoprolol 116
Microwave safety 109
Microwaved food 108
Microwaving
  and food poisoning 121
Microwaving foods
  heat-susceptor packaging
    polyethylene terpthalate
    (PET) 108
Migraine head-
    ache 155, 172
  and aspirin 178
  aspirin therapy 246
  serotonin 179
Miles Nervine Nighttime
    Sleep-Aid 111
Milk
  and cataracts 171
Minerals 191, 269
  alcoholism 278
  calcium
    absorption of 275

timed-release
    forms 276
  capsules
    absorption of 276
  iron
    immune system 279
    liver 293
  liquid forms
    absorption of 276
  multi-minerals
    absorption of 276
  potassium
    intestinal cancer 282
    sources of 282
  selenium
    deficiency 272
    natural sources of 274
    side effects 275
  timed- or slow-release
    tablets
    absorption of 276
  vinegar test
    absorption of 275
Minoxidil 123
Miscarriage 161
Misoprostol 126
Mixed incontinence
  symptoms of 257
Mixing drugs 120
Mobility
  exercise 2
Monounsaturated fatty
    acids 189
Morning sickness
  effects of ginger 97
Motion sickness
  effects of ginger 97

Mouthwash
   contact dermatitis 226
Multiple Risk Factor Inter-
      vention Trial 157
Muscle damage
   vitamin E 288
Muscle tremors 174
Muscular stress
   vitamin E 288
Myeloid leukemia
   vitamin A treatment 276

N

Nail damage
   selenium 275
Nail polish
   contact dermatitis 226
Napping
   and insomnia 236
Natural body rhythms 38
Nausea 10, 125, 155
   effects of ginger 97
   selenium 275
Nerve damage 171
Nerve disorders 104
Nerve growth factor 7
Nervous system
   damage to
      selenium 275
   vitamin B 12 171
Niacin 57. *See also Vita-*
      mins
   as a drug 272
   cholesterol 272
   liver damage 270
   nicotinic acid 271
      diabetics 272

side effects
   itching 271
slow-release forms 270
sustained-release tab-
      lets 270
Nicotine
   gum 52. *See also*
      Smoking
   withdrawal 51
Nicotine gum
   effects of acidic foods and
      drinks 127
   saliva acidity 127
Nicotinic acid 271, 272
Nitrogen dioxide 166
Nonsteroidal anti-inflam-
      matory drug (NSAID)
      therapy 118
Nonsteroidal anti-inflam-
      matory drugs
   internal bleeding 119
NutraSweet
   orange juice diet
      weight loss 292
Nutrition 191
   and drugs 133
Nutritional problems
   and taste 129
Nytol tablets 111. *See*
      also Sleep problems

O

Oat bran
   glucans 201
Oat bran extract 200
   oatrim 200
Obesity
   sleep apnea 239

Oil glands
  skin problems
    dry skin 232
Olive oil 189
Omega-3
    fish oil 17, 34, 195,
    197. *See also Fish oil*
  effects on breast
    cancer 34
  protects against
    cancer 64
Oral contraceptives
  urinary tract
    infections 254
Orange juice diet
  weight loss 291. *See
    also Diet*
Osteoarthritis 10, 11,
    12. *See also Arthritis*
Osteoclasts 214
Osteoporosis 1, 13, 170,
    211. *See also Brittle-
    bone disease*
  and caffeine 216
  and gum disease 215
  and teeth 170
  and tooth decay 215
  brittle bone disease 1
  fluoride treatment 215
Ovarian cancer 105. *See
    also Cancer*
Ovaries 185
Overflow incontinence
  symptoms of 257
Overweight
  jogging 144
Oxidation 190
  vitamin E 288

P

Pain relief 172
Painting
  and mercury poison-
    ing 174
Pancreas 24
  insulin 24
Pancreatic cancer
  selenium
    deficiency 273. *See
    also Cancer*
Paralysis 48
Parathyroid hormones 213
Parkinson's disease
  pain relief
    aspirin in lotion 226
Parrot fever 161
Paxipam 103
Pelvic inflammatory dis-
    ease 156
Pelvic swelling 125
Peptic ulcers 100. *See
    also Ulcers*
  and Helicobacter pylori
    bacteria 100
Perfume
  contact dermatitis 226
Pernicious anemia
  vitamin B12 defi-
    ciency 281
Personality changes 176
Pets 159
  parasite 160
  roundworm
    toxicare Canis 160
  toxoplasmosis 160
  zoonoses 159

Phenols 63
Phlebitis 261
  deep-vein 262
  prevention tips 262
Phosphorus 133, 205. *See
  also Minerals*
Physical handicaps
  urinary inconti-
    nence 257
Phytosterolemia 124
Plant sterols 124
Plants
  contact dermatitis 226
Plaque
  build-up in arteries
    vitamin C 280
Plasma
  selenium deficiency 274
Platelets 196
  and migraine head-
    aches 178
Pneumonia 60, 202
Poison 174
Poison ivy
  skin problems 228
Poison oak
  skin problems 228
Poison sumac
  skin problems 228
Pollutants 143
Pollution 166
Polycythemia vera
  pruritus 265
Polycythemia vera 264
  bloodshot eyes 265
  intestinal hemor-
    rhages 265

risk of thrombosis 265
symptoms of 265
ulcers 265
Polymyalgia 123
Polyunsaturated fatty
  acids 74
Polyunsaturated vegetable
  oils 206
Postmenopause
and loss of
    calcium 211. *See also
    Menopause*
Potassium 21, 133. *See
  also Minerals*
anti-stroke effects 21
blood pressure 25
blood pressure reducing
  effects 21
intestinal cancer 282
protects heart 25
ratio to sodium
  cancer protection 282
sources of 26, 282
Preeclampsia 81
Premature births 161
Premenstrual symptoms
Seasonal Affective
  Disorder 219
Processed foods
cancer-causing chemicals
  vitamin C 282
Progestin 185
and cholesterol 185
Propranolol 114, 116
Prostaglandins 118
Protease inhibitor 87
Protein 76, 193

cholesterol 76
and kidney damage 197
Pruritus
polycythemia vera 265
Psittacosis
symptoms 161
Psoriasis 196, 227. *See
also Skin problems*
vitamin D cream 230
Psychiatric problems
sleeping disorders
sleeping pills 238
Psyllium 77, 203
allergic reactions 78
and oat bran 203
flea wort 204
Puffy eyes 168
Pulse 14, 140

Q

Quinine 166

R

Rabies 163
Radical
mastectomy 34. *See
also Breast cancer*
Rash
and urinary
incontinence 256. *See
also Skin problems*
contact dermatitis 224
Raynaud's disease 265
simple treatment 265
Red blood cells
anemia

vitamin B12 defi-
ciency 281
liver 293
Renal activity 118
Respiratory
problems 161. *See
also Breathing problems*
Rest
and chronic heart fail-
ure 187
Retin-A 125
Retina 148
Retinoic acid
leukemia treatment 276
Rheumatoid arthritis 9,
10, 17, 18. *See also
Arthritis*
and omega-3 fatty
acids 196
Riboflavin
vegetarian diet 277. *See
also Vitamins*
Rice bran 169
Ringworm
symptoms of 161
Rocky mountain spotted
fever
symptoms 162

S

Salicylism 122
Saliva 154
Salmonella 121
symptoms of 163
Salt
stroke 266, 267
Saturated fat 189, 275

Saunas
  and dry skin 224
Scurvy 20
Seasonal Affective Disor-
    der 217
  sleep disturbances 219
Secondary smoke 142
  vitamin E 277
Sedatives 103
Seizures 104, 153
Selenium 31, 64, 191,
    272. *See also Minerals*
  natural sources of 274
  protects against
    cancer 64
  side effects 275
Self-esteem 4, 5
Senility 153
  sleep apnea 240
Serax 103
Serotonin 179
Sexual impotence
  drug side effects
    weight loss 296
Sexual performance
  vitamin E 288
Shift workers
  Seasonal Affective Disor-
    der 219
Shingles
  skin pain relief
    aspirin in lotion 226
Sick building syndrome
  symptoms of 120
Silver fillings 173
Skin disease 161
Skin odor
  selenium 275

Skin problems 221
  aging 232
  allergic skin reac-
    tion 228
  and liver disease 231
  contact dermatitis 224
    among the elderly 233
    common causes 225
    treatments 233
  dry skin 221
    alcoholic drinks 222
    caffeinated drinks 222
    cosmetics 223
    diabetes mellitus 222
    moisturizing lo-
      tions 222
    "soak-grease"
      method 222
    tepid bath 232
    Xerosis 232
  in the elderly 232
    sweat glands 232
  insect stings
    allergic reaction 229
  itching
    lichen planus 231
    niacin 271
  jaundice
    liver problems 293
  lichen planus
    and liver disease 231
  lichen simples
    chronicus 233
  pruritus
    polycythemia vera 265
  psoriasis 227
    vitamin D cream 230
  rash 228

contact dermatitis 224
shingles
  pain relief 226
skin color
  polycythemia vera 264
skin flushing
  niacin 271
skin odor
  selenium 275
tinged skin
  beta carotene 286
tuliposide
  allergic reaction 231
urinary inconti-
  nence 256
Skin rash 167, 176
Skin tags 85
Skipped heartbeats 142
Sleep 168
Sleep apnea
  alcohol 242
  Alzheimer's disease 240
  and dementia 240
  and snoring 239
  caffeine 242
  exercise 242
  helpful tips 241
  medications 241
  obesity 239
  sleep problems
    treatments 238
  smoking 239
  snoring
    helpful tips 240
  surgery 240
  weight loss 239
Sleep clinics
  and insomnia 236

Sleep disturbances
  Seasonal Affective Disor-
    der 219
Sleep problems 235
  anxiety
    sleeping pills 238
  hide serious disor-
    ders 237
  insomnia 235
    causes 235
    helpful tips 236
  psychiatric problems
    sleeping pills 238
  shift workers
    body clock 243
  skimping on sleep
    consequences 238
    gastrointestinal dis-
    eases 239
    heart ailments 239
    shorten life span 238
  sleep apnea
    alcohol 242
    Alzheimer's dis-
    ease 240
    caffeine 242
    dementia 240
    exercise 242
    helpful tips 241
    medications 241
    obesity 239
    smoking 239
    snoring 239
    treatments 238
    weight 239
  sleep clinics 236
  stress
    sleeping pills 238

Sleep-eze 3 111
Sleepinal Night-time Sleep
    Aid 111
Sleeping medication
    and insomnia 237
Sleeping pills 103
    over-prescribed 237
Slurred speech 174
Smoking 48, 50, 137,
    157. *See also Breathing
    problems*
    and cardiovascular
        disease 190
    and risk of
        osteoporosis 215
    depression from
        smoking 51
    effects of caffeine 56
    effects on anemia 52
    healing process 53
    heart attack 50
    heart damage 49
    sleep apnea 239
    ways to stop 53
Sneezing
    stress incontinence 256
Snoring
    sleep apnea
        helpful tips 240
Snuff 154
Sodium
    ratio to potassium
        cancer protection 282
Sodium ascorbate
    immune system 279
Sodium fluoride 215
    and osteoporisis 215
Sodium retention 134

Sodium-bicarbonate 134
Sominex 111
Sominex Pain Relief for-
    mula 111
Sores
    urinary inconti-
        nence 256
South American lily
    poisonous plants 231
Soybean extract
    and liver damage 208
Soybean lecithin 209
Soybeans
    isoflavones
        effects on cancer 41
Starches
    sources of 84
Steam baths
    and dry skin 224
Stomach
    vitamin and mineral
        absorption 275
Stomach cancer
    selenium
        deficiency 273. *See
        also Cancer*
Stomachache 119
Storing medications 121
Stress 109, 204
    and caffeine 109
    and cancer 204
    and insomnia 235
    muscular
        vitamin E 288
    sleeping problems
        sleeping pills 238
Stress diet 205

Stress incontinence 256
  symptoms of 256
Stroke 21, 48, 73, 104,
  124, 135
  aspirin therapy 245,
  246
  atherosclerosis
    vitamin C 280
  beta carotene 286
  brain tissue damage
    dietary salt 267
  effects of smoking 48
  medications
    inhibit recovery 247
  thrombosis
    polycythemia vera 265
  tissue plasminogen
    activator
    blood clots 264
  vitamin B 269
Sugar 30
  effects on cancer 30
  fructose
    orange juice diet 291
  glucose
    orange juice diet 291
Sulfur dioxide 64
Sunshine
  Seasonal Affective Disor-
    der 217
Sweat glands
  skin problems
    in the elderly 232
Sweating 176
Swelling
  insect bites
    allergic reactions 229

Swimmer's ear 158
  otitis externa 158
Swimming 11
Swimming pools
  and urinary tract infec-
    tions 254

T

Tampons
  contact dermatitis 226
Target heart rate 13, 140
Tea
  and osteoporosis 216
Teeth loss 170, 215
Tetracyclines 134
Thiamin
  vegetarian diet 277. See
    also Vitamins
Thiazide diuretics 116
Thiotepa 105
Thrombosis
  polycythemia vera 265
Thyroid gland 97
Thyroid problems 249
  over and under ac-
    tive 249
Thyroiditis 97
Timed-release forms
  calcium
    absorption of 276
Timolol 152
Tin 173
Tissue plasminogen activa-
    tor 135, 141
  dissolves blood
    clots 263

Tobacco smoke
  free radicals
    vitamin C   281
Tooth fillings   173
Toothpaste
  contact dermatitis   226
Toxicare Canis
  symptoms of   160
Toxoplasmosis
  symptoms of   160
TPA. *See Tissue plasmino-*
    gen activator
Tranquilizers   103
Trans fatty acids   207
  hydrogenation   207
Tranxene   103
Trazodone   104
  side effects   104
Treosulfan   105
Tretinoin   125
Triglycerides   196, 197
Triprolidine   111
Tuliposide
  South American lily
    allergic reaction   231
Tumor   30, 31,
    33, 37, 66, 85
  intestinal
    potassium   282
Tumor-like growths   124
Turmeric
  curcumin effects on
    cancer
    sources of   66
Tylenol   124

U

Ulcer   97, 126

  effects of tea and
    coffee   97
Ulcer disease   101, 126
Ulcers   119
  antacids   119
  effects of ginger   97
  polycythemia vera   265
Ultraviolet light   161
Unsaturated fats   207
Urea   123
Uric acid   57
Urinary
  incontinence   256. *See*
    also Incontinence
  at-home remedies   257
  different types   256
  drug therapy   257
  functional incontinence
    symptoms of   257
  mixed incontinence   257
  overflow incontinence
    symptoms of   257
  stress incontinence
    symptoms of   256
  surgery   257
  urge incontinence
    symptoms of   256
Urinary tract infection
  causes and
    symptoms. *See also*
      Kidneys
Urinary tract infections
  kidney damage   256
  menopause   253
Urine   154

V

Vaginal bleeding   125
Vaginal canal   156
Valium   103, 130
Varicose veins
  and phlebitis   262
Vascular and circulation
    problems
  blood clots
    cholesterol   263
  fibrin
    blood clots   263
    heart disease   263
  phlebitis
    prevention tips   262
  polycythemia vera   264
    heart attacks   265
    intestinal hemor-
      rhages   265
    risk of thrombosis   265
    symptoms of   265
    ulcers   265
  Raynaud's disease   265
    simple treatment   265
  salt
    brain tissue dam-
      age   266
  stroke
    dietary salt   266
  tissue plasminogen
    activator
    dissolves blood
      clots   263
  vitamin E
    atherosclerosis preven-
      tion   267

Vascular and circulatory
    problems
  hardening of the arteries
    vitamin E   267. *See
    also Atherosclerosis*
  phlebitis
    blood clots   261
Vascular disease   89
Vasculitis   16
Vegetables   28
  cruciferous
    cancer-fighting
      effects   29
    effects on breast
      cancer   28
Vegetarians   33
  vitamin deficiencies   277
Vinegar test   275
Vitamin A   64, 83, 124,
    133, 192
  deficiency of
    hearing loss   283
  leukemia treatment   276
  protects against can-
    cer   64
  retinoic acid
    leukemia treat-
      ment   277
  vegetarian diet   277
Vitamin B   269
  artherosclerosis   269
  folate
    deficiency of   281
  hyperhomo-
    cysteinemia   269
  risk of stroke   269
Vitamin B-complex   124

Vitamin
   B12   171, 192, 270
   and vegetarian diet   277
   cobalamin
      deficiency of   281
   deficiency of
      leukemia   281
   natural sources of   282
Vitamin B3
   liver failure   270
Vitamin B6   192, 270
   vegetarian diet   277
Vitamin B9
   deficiency of
      leukemia   281
Vitamin
   C   19, 57, 124, 150, 201
   alcohol detoxifica-
      tion   278
   and smokers   191
   antioxidant
      free radicals   280
   breast cancer protec-
      tion   32
   cholesterol
      build-up in arter-
      ies   280
   deficiency of
      scurvy   20
   immune system   279
   natural sources of   280
      cramping   20
      diarrhea   20
      gout   20
      kidney stones   20
   processed foods
      cancer-causing chemi-
      cals   280

sodium ascorbate
   immune system   279
Vitamin D   64, 80,
   82, 133, 213
   and bone loss   213
   and osteoporosis   214
   and psoriasis   230
   and vegetarian diet   277
   protects against can-
      cer   64
   sources of   80, 205
Vitamin D3
   calcitriol   230
Vitamin deficiencies
   and food taste   129
Vitamin E   31, 53,
   64, 133, 150
   alcohol   289
   selenium
      antioxidants   274
   anemia   288
   arteries
      cholesterol build-
      up   280
   atherosclero-
      sis   267, 284, 288
   atherosclerosis
      therapy   267
   blood clots   288
   cholesterol   288
   deficiency   288
   drug abuse   288
   effects on smoking   53
   energy
      lack of   288
   exercise
      muscle damage   288

hyperthyroidism 288
immune system 288
irritability 288
muscle weakness
  muscle damage 288
natural sources of 288
oxidation 288
protects against
  cancer 64
secondary smoke 277
sexual performance 288
vegetarian diet 277
Vitamin K 191
Vitamin-mineral supple-
  ments 191
Vitamins 171, 269
alcoholism 278
and cataracts 150
antioxidant 280
  vitamin E 274, 284
beta carotene
  heart problems 286
  sources of 286
  tinged skin 286
capsules
  absorption of 276
carotenoid compounds
  sources of 286
cobalamin
  leukemia 281
cooking and can-
  ning 282
deficiency of
  immune system 285
effects of heat 282
exercise
  muscle damage 288

folate
  deficiency of 281
  natural sources of 281
  vegetarian diet 277
generic-brand multi-
  vitamins
  absorption of 276
hearing loss
  vitamin A defi-
  ciency 283
immune system
  aging process 285
liquid forms
  absorption of 276
liver storage 293
niacin 272
  liver damage 270
  nicotinic
  acid 271, 272
previtamin A
  heart problems 285
protection against atherosclerosis 284
riboflavin
  vegetarian diet 277
slow-release forms 270
sodium ascorbate
  immune system 279
sustained-release tab-
  lets 270
thiamin
  vegetarian diet 277
timed- or slow-release
  tablets
  absorption of 276
vinegar test
  absorption of 275

Vomiting 95

W

Walkers 12
Walking 10, 12, 22, 136, 172
  and a healthy heart 138
  and tissue plasminogen
    activator 141
Walking tips 138
Warfarin
  anti-stroke therapy 245
Warts
  removal
    side effects 231
Water pills
  sexual impotence
    weight loss 296
Water retention 134
Weakness 171
  polycythemia vera 265
Weight
  ideal weight 296
  losing weight 10
Weight gain
  and Seasonal Affective
    Disorder 219
  propranolol 114
Weight lifting 1, 2
Weight
  loss 22, 168, 291, 293
  appetite
    orange juice diet 291
  aspartame 291
  calories
    dieting 295
    orange juice diet 291
  coronary disease 294

diet
  liver health 293
dieting
  metabolic rate 295
diuretics
  sexual impotence 296
exercise 295
  liver health 293
gout 294
heart 292
heart disease 294
high-fiber cereals 72
hypertension
  sexual impotence 296
ideal weight 293
liver 293
metabolic rate 297
phlebitis 262
sexual impotence 296
sleep apnea 239
water pills
  sexual impotence 296
Whirlpools 11
Wine
  and insomnia 236
Winter depression
  Seasonal Affective Disor-
    der 218
Wood's lamp 161
Wrinkle cream 125

X

Xanax 103
Xerosis
  skin problems 232

Z

Zinc   134, 193. *See also*
   Minerals
Zoonoses   159. *See also*
   Pets